The Asthma and Allergy Action Plan for Kids

A COMPLETE PROGRAM TO HELP YOUR CHILD LIVE A FULL AND ACTIVE LIFE

Allen J. Dozor, M.D.
AND Kate Kelly

A FIRESIDE BOOK
Published by Simon & Schuster
New York   London   Toronto   Sydney

FIRESIDE
Rockefeller Center
1230 Avenue of the Americas
New York, NY 10020

FIRESIDE and colophon are registered trademarks
of Simon & Schuster, Inc.

Designed by Christine Weathersbee

Manufactured in the United States of America

10   9   8   7   6   5   4   3   2   1

Library of Congress Cataloging-in-Publication Data
Allergies and asthma action plan for kids: a complete program to
help your child live a full and active life/ Allen J. Dozor and Kate
Kelly.
p. cm.
Includes bibliographical references.
1. Allergy in children. 2. Allergy in children—Prevention.
3. Allergy in children—Patients—Care. 4. Asthma in children.
5. Asthma in children—Prevention. 6. Asthma in children—Patients—Care. I. Kelly, Kate. II. Title.
RJ386.D696 2004
618.92'97—dc22

                      2003063514

ISBN 0-7432-3577-0

For information regarding special discounts for bulk
purchases, please contact Simon & Schuster Special Sales
at 1-800-456-6798 or business@simonandschuster.com.

This publication contains the opinions and ideas of its authors. It is intended to provide helpful and informative material on the subjects addressed in the publication. It is sold with the understanding that the authors and publisher are not engaged in rendering medical, health, or any kind of personal professional services in the book. The reader should consult his or her medical, health, or other competent professional before adopting any of the suggestions in this book or drawing inferences from it.

The authors and the publisher specifically disclaim all responsibility for any liability, loss, or risk, personal or otherwise, which is incurred as a consequence, directly or indirectly, of the use and application of any of the contents of this book.

CONTENTS

INTRODUCTION:

Why This Book Is
So Important to Me

Soon after I began working in medical research as part of a summer science program in high school, I knew that I loved academic medicine. Clinical research seemed a great way of combining my desire to do something "important" with the joy of learning. I devoted most summers in high school and college to cardiac and cardiovascular research, and I seemed destined for a career as an academic cardiologist. But in my pediatric residency in New York City, I learned that the number one reason children were hospitalized was respiratory disease. For three years I worked more than a hundred hours a week caring for children with difficulty breathing. I was struck by how little we really understood about common childhood illnesses such as allergies and asthma, croup, bronchitis, pneumonia, and cystic fibrosis; and how often our medications proved inadequate. I remember doing everything I could for a child and then sitting with anxious parents, all of us praying their child would get better.

It's hard to believe now, but back then there were no specialists for these most common illnesses in pediatrics—there were no pediatric pulmonologists. When I learned that a few of the major children's hospitals in the country had small training programs, including Harvard's Children's Hospital in Boston, a lightbulb went on for me. Here was an opportunity to do something new and special and very important.

I was fortunate to have excellent pediatricians, who were really good at taking care of children with breathing problems, as role models. With their guidance, I cared for hundreds of children with asthma and watched many patients of all ages die of respiratory failure—from two-pound babies in the neonatal ICU to teenagers and young adults with cystic fibrosis. As a resident I often stayed up all night at the bedside of a child gasping for air. I remember like it was yesterday an eight-year-old with severe croup, a disease that normally affects infants and toddlers. With croup, anxiety and fear significantly worsen respiratory distress, so I spent the night holding this boy's hand and reassuring him to keep him calm. By the time the sun came up the next morning, the medicines had taken effect. His breathing relaxed at last. I felt exhilarated; we had made it through together.

Children are so wonderful, so innocent and fresh, so trusting and appreciative. No matter how tired I was after one of those thirty-six-hour shifts, I would saunter home feeling so lucky that these children and their parents allowed me to share these special moments with them. I continue to pursue solutions for these children; and I have made my life's work caring for youngsters who suffer from all types of breathing difficulties. While much of this information is applicable to adults, my area of expertise is children. If your child with allergies or asthma is older than twenty-one, this is not the book for you.

I have written this book to empower parents not to settle

for less than optimal control of their child's allergies or asthma. Parents have the right to demand more from their physicians and from the medications they prescribe. I want to convey this message to as many parents as possible so our children grow up living happy, active lives.

Allen J. Dozor, M.D.

August 2003

PART ONE:

WHAT IS HAPPENING TO YOUR CHILD?

ONE

An Unnecessary Burden: Feeling Fair-to-Poor When Good-to-Great Is Possible

Allergies and asthma are two of the fastest growing health problems for children, and their complexity challenges both doctors and parents. What causes a rash or mild wheezing in one youngster may cause another to be hospitalized. Lunchtime, a birthday party, or a school trip can be life-threatening for a child with severe food allergies. Allergies to insects or drugs can be medical emergencies. A child's allergies or asthma affects everyone around them: parents, teachers, coaches, baby-sitters, and even schoolmates.

Every day I meet parents desperate for information: What is asthma? What are allergies? What's the difference between croup, bronchitis, asthma, and pneumonia? Will our child grow out of it? Do we need to keep our children on medications? What are the risks? How can we prevent an attack from occurring? Should we get rid of the cat? Can we get a dog or bird? Should we move to Arizona? What about homeopathic remedies? Would acupuncture help? Should we buy an air purifier?

Some of the most upsetting effects of allergies and asthma are the wounds these chronic conditions may inflict on a child's self-image and self-esteem: constant concern and protectiveness from parents and teachers; confusing limits and rules to follow; chronic symptoms such as fatigue, headaches, obesity, shortness of breath, itchy eyes, nasal congestion, poor sleep, chest pains, or stomachaches; and the inevitable comparisons children make to the unencumbered lives of siblings and friends. These issues all contribute to a child's feeling that he is unwell, less able to succeed in life. These symptoms may lead to a vicious cycle of inactivity, poor physical conditioning, poor sleep quality, and the embarrassment of poor athletic and academic performance. All of this is usually unnecessary.

Not Sick but Not Well Either . . .

Children with allergies or asthma may not necessarily look sick, but they aren't well either—you may know the look from your own child. These kids just don't feel "perfect." Maybe they are just sluggish, yawning more than they should. Their color may be a bit off; maybe their eyes are puffy or red, not as bright. Maybe they have "raccoon" eyes or look like they didn't get enough sleep. Maybe they have chapped lips from chronic mouth breathing, or bad breath from chronic nasal or sinus congestion. Children with poorly controlled allergies or asthma may have decreased appetites, abdominal cramps, constipation, or irregularity.

Few people—even those closest to them—realize how often children with asthma and allergies find their lives significantly altered. While severe illnesses, late-night visits to the emergency room, or hospitalizations are rarely forgotten, less obtrusive illnesses often are. "Malady amnesia" sets in; once the discomfort passes, memory fades. After about six months, many parents forget when their child came home early from school. A parent may remember writing a note to excuse Susie from gym class, but be a bit hazy about what she told them happened during recess. Many parents don't know if their child coughs frequently while sleeping. If allergies and asthma run in the family, everyone may be coughing, and parents may have become used to it. And of course, if there are two or more children in the house, memories blur.

Studies show that parents, physicians, and children often underestimate the frequency and severity of children's symptoms. Consider these one-year statistics from "Asthma in America," a recent national study conducted by the pharmaceutical company GlaxoSmithKline:

- 32% of children with asthma went to the emergency room for asthma.
- 9% of people with asthma required hospitalization for asthma.
- 29% of people with asthma had unscheduled asthma-related visits to their doctor's office or clinic.
- 49% of children with asthma missed school because of their asthma.
- 30% of patients with asthma are awakened from sleep with breathing problems at least once a week.
- Only 22% whose symptoms are consistent with severe asthma actually describe their symptoms as severe.

Most patients overestimate how well controlled their asthma actually is. Chronic low-level difficulties such as mild sneezing or coughing frequently go unaddressed, yet over time can be quite debilitating. That stuffed-up congested feeling can make it difficult for a child to function at an optimum level, whether it's sitting still for story hour in kindergarten or taking an oral French exam in high school.

Allergies or asthma can significantly interfere with participation in sports, school trips, physical education classes, and play activities. They might not sleep as deeply, or dream adequately. They may not awake fully rested. They may not be as alert or have a normal attention span. Peer relations may suffer. They might not do as well on tests and other school activities. Teachers, counselors, and administrators may notice behavioral problems or that a child's school performance has slipped.

Obesity and Asthma

Both obesity and asthma are occurring with increasing frequency, and no one is sure why. Clearly there is a relationship between these two serious problems. Kids with poorly controlled asthma are more likely to be overweight, and it is more difficult to control asthma in kids who are obese. Good asthma control may help kids exercise more and burn more calories, which would help decrease obesity.

Worrying About Life-Threatening Allergic Reactions

Severe illness is more obvious. Those with more serious forms of asthma may have been recently hospitalized or they may be going through a spell when they cough all night, depriving them of sleep and terrifying anxious parents.

These problems ripple through a community, affecting life in the classroom and at friends' homes. Is a classroom rabbit worsening a child's allergies? What about Grandma's cat? Can a child safely attend summer camp? I hear these worries every day.

Parents of children with food allergies live with a special burden. Every day they wake up and go to sleep worrying that they will slip up, that their child will eat something cooked in peanut oil, for example, and experience a life-threatening emergency.

Allergies to insect stings or latex may cause severe reactions, even anaphylactic shock. These parents find they must live a life of hypervigilance.

I remember Rachel, a teenager whose mother lived in deadly fear that her child would be exposed to peanuts. For fear that the smell from someone's bag of peanuts would take her daughter's life, Rachel's mom never allowed her to fly. And despite the fact that most airlines have responded to these concerns by banning peanuts, Rachel's parents still have not overcome their fears. My heart goes out to families who must live with these fears. My goal is to do whatever I can to lessen their burden.

Living with a Chronic Condition

One of the most difficult parts of living with allergies and asthma is coming to grips with their chronic nature—they are an "always" affair. Most childhood illnesses come and go, with an end in sight. Allergies and asthma worries never seem to end—sometimes on the front burner, sometimes on the back, but always there. This is very tiring for children, their parents, their siblings, their friends, and even for their physicians.

It gets to the point where parents don't even complain when their children fall asleep in school because of their medications, have nosebleeds from their nose sprays, or seem jittery from their inhalers. Many children and their families are accustomed to living with these chronic discomforts as well as low-level nasal stuffiness, itching, rashes, coughing, and fatigue—they're just not a "ten." Maybe they're a "nine," or sometimes an "eight." Not enough families speak up when their child coughs or wheezes after running the mile run in gym. Physicians often don't ask and parents often don't tell them that their child wakes up in the middle of the night because they can't breathe through their nose or need their inhaler. In fact, many children don't even tell their parents.

This level of discomfort is unnecessary. With attention and persistence, solutions can be found. I have heard from countless families over the years about the remarkable changes they see in their children when their symptoms are well controlled. Their children simply feel better. They sleep better, eat better, and participate more fully in family life, school, and activities with friends. Parents often notice their children are in a better mood, fighting less with their siblings, complaining less as they head off to school.

The Problem with the Do-It-Yourself Route

Seeking scheduled professional medical care is difficult, expensive, and time-consuming. Everyone is so busy it is quite understandable when a mother or father decides to run to the nearest drugstore for an over-the-counter (OTC) remedy that might offer some relief. This can be very confusing, since there are literally hundreds of medications for respiratory symptoms. Well-known brand names are often attached to many different products. For instance, let's say you're advised to give your child Robitussin, one of the most well-respected and established brands. Should you buy Robitussin expectorant, Robitussin DM, or Robitussin Cough and Cold? Should you choose regular strength or extra strength? When should you choose the "children's versions" as opposed to the regular ones? And now they all come honey flavored? What would you guess is in Robitussin Honey Flu? (Not the flu, I trust.)

These products may include any number of ingredients, in

a bewildering array of strengths, and are designed to help some or all of the common symptoms: itching, sneezing, nasal congestion, coughing, wheezing, fever, or body pains. OTC remedies are often short-acting, have limited effectiveness, and may cause side effects. A parent would never give a child a sleeping pill before sending him off to school. Yet when administering over-the-counter allergy/cold remedies, parents have often done almost the same thing—the poor kids are lucky to be able to keep their eyes open, let alone focus on the classroom lesson until 3 P.M.

One of the ironies of our American healthcare system is that many of the older over-the-counter medications may actually have more side effects than newer medications available only by prescription.

One striking example of the complexity of this situation involves the most common allergy remedies, antihistamines. The first generation of antihistamines, now more than twenty years old, was a great advance, and these medications remain important. An old-fashioned first-generation antihistamine is still the best choice during a severe acute allergic reaction. However, because these medications are short-acting and may cause drowsiness, delayed reaction time, and a dry mouth, the pharmaceutical industry has worked hard at improving on them, successfully developing second-, third-, and even now fourth-generation antihistamines with fewer side effects and longer durations of action. These advances are great for people with chronic allergies.

One of these newer antihistamines, loratidine (Clariten), is now available without prescription, which is great for many people who only need such a medication once in a while. However, these newer medications are expensive, and as long as they require a prescription, they are covered by most U.S. health insurance plans. Once they become nonprescription, the money to pay for them comes directly out of consumers' pockets. Not surprisingly, insurance companies have been vocal advocates of this "improved" access to newer medications, but consumer advocates or patients who need these medications for months or years are not so happy with this shift in expense.

Whether the best medicine for your child is prescription or over-the-counter or some combination of the two, it is still advisable to consult a doctor.

Looking for Natural Cures

More and more parents come to my office looking for natural cures, and I don't blame them. We all want to offer our children a cure that will help while causing no harm. Alternative approaches to allergies and asthma appear at a dizzying rate. Homeopathic remedies, herbal medicines, vitamin and mineral therapies, etc. have taken over huge sections of our pharmacies, health food stores, and supermarkets.

Very few of these approaches have been proven to be either effective or ineffective, because the industries profiting from these approaches are quite happy to remain in the shadows, away from the prying eyes of the FDA and other regulatory agencies. Does this mean these natural remedies don't help? No. But can you believe the claims on these packages? Sadly, this answer is also no.

The massive amount being spent on these products is a testament to the sad state of affairs for many children with allergies and asthma. Parents are rightly concerned about side effects of medications and yet they really don't want their kids to suffer, so they will try anything for their children.

Prescription medicines are getting better and better, and the side effects are also being reduced. The best approach for any family is to work with a medical professional to find the right combination that helps your child with few, if any, side effects.

In the Doctor's Office

My job is to evaluate children referred from other physicians: pediatricians, family physicians, and allergists. These are kids who are not doing well, children who have not responded adequately to their physician's approach. I see children who are coughing, sneezing, and wheezing despite many visits to many different physicians.

Every week I meet patients who are suffering needlessly: infants who have already been hospitalized once or twice; kids missing school twenty or more days each year; athletes who have given up sports; teenagers who wake up sneezing and coughing two hours earlier than necessary and are already suffering from a headache. I meet children of all ages used to jitteriness, sleepiness, and stomach pains from their medications.

Primary care physicians usually refer these children to me because they are concerned something is being missed, that they must suffer from something other than just allergies or asthma. And indeed my first goal is to make sure they don't suffer from rarer conditions. About 5 to 10 percent of children thought to have difficult-to-control allergies and asthma do turn out to have a complicating or modifying condition. The vast majority of the time, however, there is no underlying rare diagnosis. Most of the time the problem is not the diagnosis, it is the prescribed therapy that has proved inadequate.

There are many reasons for this failure to adequately control children's symptoms. It's not easy. It can be very time-consuming to manage these conditions. There is a lot of "trial and error" involved, and every child ends up requiring a slightly different approach. Then, just when you think you have a child figured out, he changes.

Pediatricians and family physicians are usually not at fault in these circumstances. The doctor who is seeing your child for a general checkup is rarely able to devote as much time focusing on one issue as a specialist can. And it is difficult for a nonspecialist to keep up with the explosion of new medications, not just for allergies and asthma, but the entire array of health conditions seen in children. Finally, as I've explained countless times, if there was one perfect medication for all children, no one would come see me!

Yet I don't believe any of these reasons is the primary explanation for why children and their families come to accept sniffling, coughing, and headaches as a way of life. To my mind, the primary difficulty is lowered expectations. Too many families have gotten used to sneezing, itching, coughing, and wheezing. This could be countered if pediatricians had the time to explain that this suffering is unnecessary. Too many patients and physicians assume that hospitalizations are to be expected, that children with asthma miss a lot of school and often require strong medications such as oral steroids.

This is not good. Allergies and asthma do not need to interfere with your children's days or their dreams. I believe that somewhere out there is a combination of medications and approaches that will allow every child to grow up feeling that the "world is their oyster." I want every child with allergies and asthma to believe they can do anything they want with their lives: climb the highest mountain, participate in any sport, aim for the Olympics if so inclined. And to not settle for side effects. I don't mean to imply that achieving this goal is easy. Temporary setbacks may be unavoidable. But these goals are attainable and well worth the effort.

I have developed a program that permits children and their

parents to successfully manage allergies and asthma and to lead a normal life. My goal is to empower families by providing the information they need.

The Importance of Family Education and Understanding

Research studies demonstrate that the more parents understand about their children's health, the better they do. With proper diagnosis (not always easy to come by) and early and aggressive treatment, allergies and asthma can be successfully managed.

I spend at least half of every appointment on education. Parents need and deserve reliable and medically sound advice. They need clear explanations, details about how allergic reactions and asthma attacks can be prevented, which medications may be helpful, and general information on how best to help their children.

The key to success is not specific drugs, but identifying goals and urging parents to always consider this question: "Is the approach we are taking meeting my child's needs?" Throughout this book I will continually ask parents to analyze and refine their goals:

Goal #1: Your child's allergies or asthma do not affect her lifestyle.

Goal #2: Your child has no significant side effects from medications.

Goal #3: Your child uses the least amount of medications to achieve goals #1 and #2.

My advice to all parents is don't settle for less. Find physicians willing to listen to you and work with you in choosing therapies that meet your needs.

Most importantly, identify specific goals of therapy for your child. To play soccer without wheezing? To wake up without a headache? To sleep through the night without coughing? These sound simple but really aren't. Parents often find it difficult to answer when I ask, "Are you happy? Is the current medical regimen working to your satisfaction?" If you address the specific issues that concern you and watch for possible side effects from any new medications, then you'll soon find a treatment plan that works.

TAKE-HOME MESSAGES

- Chronic, low-level, mild, partially controlled allergies or asthma are common and may have very significant effects on your child.

- Don't settle for inadequate control of your child's symptoms.

- Don't settle for significant side effects from medications.

- In your mind, clarify what your goals are and what you hope to achieve.

- A medical regimen does exist that can meet your and your child's needs.

- Expect your child's symptoms and medical needs to change over time.

- Find physicians who will help you determine what works best for your child.

TWO

Allergies and Asthma:
The Basics

Isaac was a bright twelve-year-old boy who came to see me after a prolonged illness. When he first became ill, his pediatrician told the family that he had bronchitis. When he returned to the office for a follow-up visit, a different doctor said, "No, this is pneumonia." Both these diagnoses were actually correct. A week later, at the third visit, a nurse practitioner told his parents that Isaac actually had asthma. This, of course, got to the heart of the matter. Because Isaac's airways (bronchial tubes) were inflamed from asthma, he couldn't quite shake the respiratory illness. At this point, Isaac was referred to me, with the goal being to prevent such prolonged illnesses in the future.

Respiratory conditions such as allergies and asthma can be very confusing, partly because they frequently blend in with other health problems, and it becomes difficult to sort them out. The more you understand about the causes and expected course of these conditions, the more confident you will feel.

Allergies and asthma have been recognized throughout the ages, and each generation of scientists have viewed these conditions differently. In the last thirty years we have seen dramatic advances in our understanding. But nature does not yield its secrets easily. The complexity of these conditions boggles the mind and has kept thousands of scientists off the streets, deep in laboratories looking for answers. We still have lots to learn, so what appears to be "fact" today will no doubt be altered by a study published tomorrow. Parents should always ask, "What's new? What other treatments should we be considering?"

Let's begin with basics. Incidentally, I have pretty bad hay fever or allergic rhinitis myself, and I frequently "forget" my medications. So I hope you don't mind if I stop to blow my nose once in a while.

Allergies: The Basics

An allergic reaction is our body's immune system on overdrive. When we are exposed to an allergen, signals flow through the body, sounding the alarm Protect Thyself. An allergic reaction is the result of this hypersensitivity. Reactions may range from sneezing or breathing difficulties to eczema and other skin reactions. (Specific allergens will be discussed in Chapter 3.)

So why does the immune system go haywire over something like a beautiful spring flower or a little cat dander? Before fully explaining this, I want to tip my hat to our immune system—one of the most amazing things about our bodies.

The immune system is basically the body's armed forces, complete with such divisions as the army, navy, marines, air force, and coast guard. Each of these specialized forces is designed for special situations, and their functions often overlap. Many battles could be fought by any one of these services; some battles require all of them. We live in a world filled with noxious stuff that could potentially harm us: viruses, bacteria, pollens, mold spores, strange foods, dust, cigarette smoke, pollution, perfume smells, animal dander, insect stings—the list could go on indefinitely. Every minute of every day we are defending ourselves, and when the system is working well, we hardly notice it. When there are irregularities in the system, however, diseases such as cancer, heart disease, and diabetes—to name just a few—may result.

Key Point: *All allergic reactions start with the production of IgE.*

IgE is a nifty little protein produced by white blood cells, and it is responsible for calling up the allergic reaction forces. We all produce this protein, but people with allergies produce more of it, more of the time. IgE then stimulates a whole host of other chemicals and cells floating around in our bloodstream, part of an orchestrated cascade of chemical reactions that result in an allergic reaction—the immune system on overdrive.

Most people who tend to have allergic reactions are called *atopic*. This means the allergic reaction force within their immune system is always on alert, ready to attack almost any protein that comes down the pike, even if simpler, less expensive defenses would have done the job. As a result, people are almost never allergic to just one substance; once the system is on alert, it's ready to go after other substances as well. An allergic reaction always occurs in response to a protein stimulus: no protein, no allergy. To trigger an allergic reaction, a person has to have had prior exposure to this stimulus—you cannot be allergic to something encountered for the first time. That's why your daughter wasn't allergic to her friend's cat on their first or second play date. Only after those first visits did her special forces decide that it never again wanted to be near a cat.

What Happens During an Allergic Reaction

An allergic reaction is a very specific type of intolerance to any foreign protein:

Environmental triggers (foreign protein)
↓
    Absorption of these proteins into the body
      ↓
        Production of IgE
         ↓
           Stimulation of a variety of cells (mast cells, eosinophils, lymphocytes)
            ↓
              Production by these cells of a "chemical cascade"
                ↓
                  Symptoms of allergies: runny nose, cough, wheeze, mucus production, rash, etc.

Reactions Vary Widely

If your child is the "allergic type," then a foreign protein placed on her skin may trigger the immediate production of IgE, which then calls in the rest of the allergic reaction force. Suddenly a rash appears, such as hives or eczema. If a child breathes in dust, IgE may be produced in the nose and wham, she's sneezing and her nose is running. If her eyes are itching, it's because something in the air, such as grass pollen or cat dander, landed on her eyes. If she is coughing or wheezing, it's because she has inhaled a protein that has triggered an IgE-mediated reaction in the bronchial tubes. You can sometimes narrow down the potential offending agents by thinking about where the reaction occurred in your child's body. Unfortunately, it isn't always easy.

To begin with, not everyone who is atopic reacts to the same proteins. One allergen may cause different reactions in different people. The family cat may cause allergic rhinitis (hay fever) in one sibling and asthma in another. The allergen (cat dander) can have an additive effect in a third child, whose mild hay fever may be exacerbated because exposure to the cat has increased her reactions to other allergens.

Another difficulty with diagnosing allergies is that symptoms and their trigger aren't always clearly connected. While sneezing every fall, wheezing after mowing the lawn, or developing hives in reaction to a perfume may be obvious, some symptoms are more difficult to tie to a specific allergen. Vague abdominal discomfort, sinus headaches, feeling like your ears are clogged, and a scratchy throat may be due to an allergy but could also be due to all sorts of other things. What about such vague constitutional symptoms as sleepiness, fatigue, shortened attention span, or moodiness? They could be due to allergic reactions, they may be from medications used to treat the allergies, they may be from a combination of both, or allergies may have nothing to do with it.

Allergies to foods or medicines are even trickier. The first part of your body that sees these allergens is your entire gastrointestinal tract, starting from the mouth and throat and all the way down to the lower intestines. You may only have symptoms limited to the GI tract, such as heartburn, abdominal cramps, gas, or diarrhea. If the offending protein, often referred to as an *antigen,* is absorbed through the intestines and into the bloodstream, then the IgE that is produced travels everywhere and may cause all kinds of problems, including rashes, difficulty breathing, joint pain, etc. The causes of these generalized, or so-called systemic, reactions are often the most difficult to diagnose and the most difficult to deal with, and they may be life-threatening.

There are still many mysteries about allergies that remain: Why do allergies fluctuate through life? What factors (biological, hormonal, environmental, and emotional) may alter how allergic someone is? How does an allergic reaction to one antigen contribute to worsening reactions to other things? Why do some people react more in their skin (hives or rashes) than in their nose or lungs? For instance, my wife developed hives when she tried Chanel #5 perfume (lucky me), and I've never had hives in my life. On the other hand, I have a terrible nose. It's kind of embarrassing in my profession, but I'm always congested. My nose overreacts to just about anything in the air. And yet, amazingly, I have never wheezed or felt "tight" in my chest.

Some reactions people think are allergies aren't really allergies at all; they are "intolerances." For instance, many people cannot tolerate cow's milk. There are many reasons for this, but by far the most common is not being able to digest the type of sugar in milk, called lactose. Lactose intolerance is not an allergy. That doesn't mean the reaction isn't a problem, but it is important to understand that food intolerance may not be an allergy and so would not be helped by allergy medications.

Allergists often see patients with a food intolerance that families fear may mean allergy. Frequent bowel movements, abdominal cramps, and gassiness may be signs of another ailment known as gluten intolerance. (Gluten is a very important protein usually derived from wheat, and it is part of most cereals and breads.) Some kids have very dramatic and severe cases of this condition, fail to gain weight, and are eventually diagnosed with this syndrome of gluten-sensitive enteropathy, also known by an old name, *celiac disease*. While this is food intolerance, not an allergy, it requires treatment because, like allergies, it can have a profound effect on a child's life.

Asthma: The Basics

Asthma is a multifaceted chronic disease that occurs when the airway passages become inflamed, making it difficult for a person to breathe. Patients say that when their asthma is untreated, it is like breathing through a straw. Asthma can be triggered by allergens, including flu and other viral infections, exercise, drugs, and many other irritants. If left untreated or poorly treated, asthma can have very significant effects on a child's long-term health. Asthma attacks sometimes require hospitalization, and deaths due to asthma have been rising steadily in recent years.

There are two important points about asthma that I will stress throughout the book. Remember them because they can make all the difference to your child:

Key Points   1. *Early aggressive treatment may lessen the severity of asthma as your child ages.*

    2. *Asthma should not be addressed just on an attack-by-attack basis. Consistent, long-term prevention and treatment is what promotes good health.*

WHAT HAPPENS WITH ASTHMA

When asthma occurs, the true problem is almost never in the lungs themselves, but in the bronchial tubes (the airways). When we breathe in, air travels down a huge system of branching tubes, a vast network that divides about twenty-six times before reaching the end. If we took our bronchial tubes and sliced them open and spread them out, they would almost cover a tennis court! This represents a far greater exposure to the outside world than our skin. Every day we breathe in thousands of gallons of air, in and out, every minute, awake or asleep, filled with almost countless numbers of particles of "stuff." Those particles are constantly bombarding the walls of our bronchial tubes. The largest particles may land in the nose or the back of the throat. If they make it past the upper airway, they might be caught up by one of the branching walls of the large airways, or *bronchi*. Smaller particles might drift down to the smallest bronchial tubes, bronchioles.

And the miracle is, if you look down the bronchial tubes of an eighty-year-old man who doesn't smoke, they look almost as clean and pink as the bronchial tubes of an infant. Where did it all go? Our outer skin is constantly getting scarred through life. I still have a small scar on my finger from whittling in Boy Scout camp. Our inner skin is better protected. We have built into our airways an extraordinarily elegant system of defenses that constantly work to protect our lungs, which, after all, must last a lifetime.

When your child's airways or bronchial tubes react to something they have breathed in, you usually can tell because he or she will cough. All humans cough, all the time, every day. An elegant and simple study was conducted in London a few years back, in which tape recorders were attached to the backs of about one hundred school-age kids with no history of respiratory illness. Every child coughed every day. We all do. We don't even realize we are doing it.

But within that group of children, there was a wide range of both the severity and frequency of their coughing. Some coughed an average of only once or twice a day. Some coughed twenty or thirty times a day. Some coughed more than a hundred times each day. Based on this and other studies, we know that there is a wide spectrum of how reactive the airways are. Everyone will react at some point to a smoky room, but those with more sensitive airways will react by coughing sooner and more strongly.

Key Point: *People with asthma have*
"hyperreactive" or more
sensitive airways.

The reaction of the bronchial tubes is quite complex and involves hundreds of chemicals and thousands of cells, but it can be simplified as *inflammation*. People with lifelong asthma almost always have a little bit of inflammation going on in their airways, even when they feel great. The amount of inflammation seems to fluctuate for all sorts of reasons. When the airways are really red and sore, they are very reactive, or "twitchy." During those times, almost anything will make your child wheeze. Other times, a child's bronchial tubes will be calm and she may tolerate the exact same trigger that made her so sick last year. Our goal is to do everything possible to calm down your child's airways.

Once a child has hyperreactive or hyperresponsive airways, many things can cause irritation. Only some of the time is that reaction truly allergic—that is, a reaction triggered by IgE directed against a foreign protein. Parents hope that there are only one or two specific triggers for their child's asthma, and that eliminating those irritants will solve the problem. Sorry. Your child's sensitive airways may be triggered by just about anything.

IDENTIFYING ASTHMA

Doctors can usually identify which part of the bronchial tree has been attacked based on the signs and symptoms. If something lands on the very largest airway, the trachea, coughing will be quite loud. There are almost no mucus glands in the trachea, so anything that irritates it will trigger a loud, dry, barking, hacking, or seal-like cough. When this suddenly occurs in infants and young children, doctors usually refer to this as *croup*, meaning the trouble is occurring high in the airways.

If a foreign substance lands deeper, in the large bronchial tubes, airways react by stimulating lots of mucus. Airways are counted in generations, with the trachea being number 1. This then divides into generations 2, 3, etc., down to 26 or so. There are lots of mucus glands in the large bronchial tubes, generations 2 through 4, so if someone has a chesty productive cough, the irritation is probably in these airways and doctors may call it *bronchitis*. To a pediatric pulmonologist, the difference between croup and bronchitis is an inch or two.

When airway generations 3 through 7 or so get irritated, difficulties start to increase. Thanks to the mathematics of branching tubes, these airways cover a very large surface area. There are fewer mucus glands, so coughing tends to be drier. But the swelling, inflammation, and spasm of the smooth muscle in the walls of these tubes can lead to significant distress. If small airways narrow slightly, kids may not even notice it or will complain of vague chest pains or discomfort. If they narrow a bit more, a child may feel short of breath or find it necessary to sigh. If they narrow still a little more, then you may actually hear wheezing as the air goes in and out. When this happens, most physicians will recognize the problem and call it asthma. And if the tubes narrow even more, allowing little or no air through those particularly inflamed small airways, then you may not hear any wheezing at all. So, sometimes a child is having a bad asthma attack and you can't even tell with a stethoscope. Fortunately, there are usually many other signs to tip everyone off.

Continuing down into the lungs, generations 7 through 10 of the bronchial tubes may also react to stuff breathed in. These airways are very narrow to start with and you can't hear the air flowing through them very easily. But if a doctor using a stethoscope listens very carefully as someone breathes, the airflow traveling through strands of mucus in airways that are opening and closing gives a sound known as "crackles," or what used to be commonly referred to by physicians as "rales." When crackles are heard, many doctors diagnose pneumonia, when this may just be another form of asthma. I hasten to add that pneumonia may also refer to an actual infection of the lungs themselves, not just in the small airways. But the majority of mild pneumonias are actually due to an asthmatic reaction in very small airways.

Every doctor and parent can figure out that a child with wheezing probably has asthma. But many are surprised to learn that most children with repeated bouts of croup, bronchitis, and pneumonia also really have asthma. The difference is just which size bronchial tubes are reacting that time.

How Allergies and Other Irritants Trigger Asthma

Asthma may be triggered by a very long list of irritants, *not* just allergies. In fact, some children who wheeze and cough a lot really don't have significant allergies. And many people

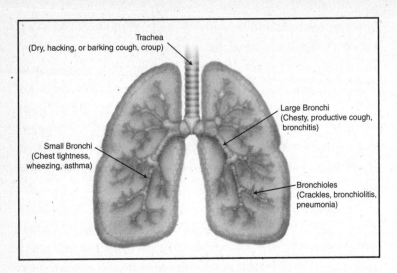

Trachea
(Dry, hacking, or barking cough, croup)

Large Bronchi
(Chesty, productive cough, bronchitis)

Small Bronchi
(Chest tightness, wheezing, asthma)

Bronchioles
(Crackles, bronchiolitis, pneumonia)

with allergies don't have asthma. But essentially all people with lifelong asthma also have allergies. Clear as mud, huh?

Respiratory infections, usually viruses, are actually responsible for the majority of severe asthma attacks in children, not allergies. Young kids have an immature immune system, and from September to June—the months when viral illnesses are more prevalent—they often catch many infections. You can eliminate every allergen in your environment and wash their hands hourly, yet your children will still catch colds. As your child's immune system matures, the number of viral infections will gradually decrease, usually dropping to just one or two each school year by the age of six to eight.

Everyone reacts to viral respiratory infections differently. Some kids may only have a stuffy nose, hardly noticeable. But then they may spread the infection to your child with asthma, and he or she may start to cough or wheeze. My two kids always caught the same colds but had their own style of suffering. My daughter's nose would stuff up, but my son would cough since he has hyperreactive airways.

If your child's asthma is triggered by both infections and

allergies, then the problem may be more chronic and more insidious. Allergies in children rarely cause the severe and dramatic attacks triggered by viral infections. But while asthma symptoms may be milder, they will occur essentially every day that your child is exposed to that specific allergen. So if your child is allergic to dust or dust mites, they will be exposed daily and may wake up coughing or wheezing every night. If your child's airways are sensitive to grass pollen, he or she may have symptoms for weeks each spring.

Exercise, particularly in cold, dry air, is also a common trigger. This will be discussed in detail in Chapter 16, but suffice it to say that this tends to occur only when kids are really running hard, huffing and puffing for at least a few minutes, rarely with mild exertion.

Wait, we're not done. Asthma may be triggered by more than just viruses, allergens, and exercise. There are lots of other irritants that may trigger a reaction from the bronchial tubes. A big problem, of course, is cigarette smoke, especially from someone else's cigarette. Many of the pollutants in cigarette smoke are in higher concentration in smoke drifting from the end of a cigarette than in the smoke inhaled directly. Then there's pollution. There are clear and reproducible increases in emergency room visits for asthma when air pollution is increased. And indoor air may be an even bigger problem than outdoor air. We have tighter windows and better insulation in our homes, our schools, and our workplaces, and our indoor air is not recirculated very often. My office is now in a beautiful new building, and I can't open the windows! While temperature control within a building is aided by tightness, this airtight system keeps all the chemicals from furniture and pressed wood and carpeting locked into our buildings, and many kids react to these indoor pollutants.

Scientists are also starting to understand that all of

these triggers cannot be viewed as separate problems; there is a synergy among them. Viral infections can increase airway reactivity to allergens, making a merely "under the weather" or sick child seem even more allergic than she really is. And allergic reactions can stimulate an increased reaction to viral infections. Kids with chronic nasal stuffiness due to allergies are much more prone to recurrent ear and sinus infections. These chronic infections are responsible for quite a bit of genuine suffering as well as many lost school days and additional visits to the doctor. If your child has asthma or hyperreactive airways, postnasal drip that often develops as part of these upper respiratory tract infections can cause an impressive amount of severe coughing. And this coughing, incidentally, is generally much more difficult to treat than straightforward asthma.

Popular Myths About Allergies and Asthma

Since allergies and asthma are common, poorly understood, and frustrating, it's not surprising that all kinds of theories have arisen to help explain these problems. As a result there are many myths that permeate our culture. And like many popular theories, there may be some hidden kernels of truth. It's important to get medical advice about the issues that concern you. For example, withholding milk from a child because "milk makes mucus" is a big mistake nutritionally. How many of the following myths have you heard? (Then see below for the truth!)

Myths About Allergies and Asthma

1. You don't have to worry about young children with asthma because they will probably outgrow it.

2. You have to wheeze to have asthma, or if you wheeze you must have asthma.

3. Asthma is mostly psychological.

4. If you have allergies you should move to Arizona.

5. Milk makes mucus, so don't let kids with allergies or asthma drink milk.

6. The most common reason for asthma is food allergies.

7. The steroids often given for asthma are the same medications illicitly used by athletes to build muscles.

8. Any side effect from a medication means you are allergic to that medication.

9. Children with asthma can't play sports.

10. Hospitalizations for asthma are inevitable.

Myth #1:
You don't have to worry about young children with asthma because they will probably outgrow it.

This myth is dangerous. Young children go from really well to really sick really fast. Ignoring chronic coughing and wheezing in young children is not a good idea. Take your child to your pediatrician and get a professional evaluation—if nothing else comes of it, your doctor can almost certainly make your child more comfortable during a specific respiratory illness.

And although many kids who cough and wheeze with respiratory infections will have a decreasing number of severe illnesses over time, most adults with asthma start wheezing as young children.

Key Point: *There is increasing evidence that early aggressive treatment of young children with asthma may actually lessen the long-term severity of this condition.*

As for allergies, they often worsen over time, and the sooner you get your child's under control, the more comfortable he or she will be.

Myth #2:
You have to wheeze to have asthma, or if you wheeze you must have asthma.

Many children and adults with asthma don't actually wheeze, or they wheeze only rarely. They may just cough a lot. Or they may develop chest congestion or shortness of breath. Some just describe chest pain or vague discomfort. Wheezing results from the narrowing of smaller airways. If your larger bronchial tubes react to a trigger, you may not wheeze at all yet still have asthma.

Incidentally, most people with hyperreactive airways don't think of themselves as having a disease or as having asthma. About 30 percent of everyone you know has increased airway reactivity. Here's a trick question: Next time you are at a party, ask everyone if they ever feel tight in the chest when they catch a cold or run long distances. If they say yes, they have hyperreactive airways. In other words, they have asthma.

Myth #3:
Asthma is mostly psychological.

Any parent of a child suffering from asthma knows this is not true. Yet kids sometimes aren't taken seriously, particularly by teachers and athletic coaches who often fear that if they exempt one or two students from an activity they'll have a lineup of kids claiming to have some condition that means that he shouldn't have to run the mile or shouldn't have to take part in the class cleanup project on Earth Day.

Asthma is undeniably a physical condition. However, psychology does play an important role in asthma. When kids get anxious during an asthma attack they breathe even faster, which in turn may actually trigger more wheezing or coughing.

The perception of asthma by children certainly varies. Ironically, some kids can have a full 25 percent narrowing of their bronchial tubes and deny even feeling it; others notice as little as a 5 percent drop. But children with asthma are not making it up.

Myth #4:
If you have allergies you should move to Arizona.

I love Arizona and who knows, maybe someday I'll move there, but not because of my allergies. If you were to take your child to a different geographical area, he might initially find relief simply because you've left behind the allergens he reacted to at home. Unfortunately, the child—or person—who is atopic will probably develop allergic reactions to the local allergens in the new environment sooner or later. Unless you are prepared to move to a different climate and geography every six months, never returning again, a household move won't work. I guess you can run, but you can't hide.

Myth #5:
Milk makes mucus, so don't let kids with allergies or asthma drink milk.

By and large this is not true. There have been at least five good studies from many countries examining this issue. In the vast majority of children and adults with allergies and asthma, there is no increase in mucus production after drinking milk. Many people get confused because milk can coat your throat, but that's it. Of course some people are truly allergic to the proteins in cow's milk, and they may react to milk with all sorts of symptoms, including increased mucus, but this is much less common than most people believe; parents need to check this out with a doctor before assuming the child is allergic to milk. For more information see Chapter 6, "Identifying Food Allergies."

Myth #6:
The most common reason for asthma is food allergies.

Almost every week I meet parents convinced their child's diet is causing asthma, so they come to me with a full analysis of their child's food intake, trying to sort out why their child's asthma seems out of control. While their efforts are well intended and some children do cough and wheeze as part of an allergic reaction to food, this is relatively uncommon. Generally speaking, allergic reactions to food will occur within an hour or so after eating, so the pattern is quite recognizable.

If allergies play a significant role in your child's asthma, then it is usually environmental allergens inhaled into their lungs. As you'll see later in the book, the search for specific allergens is well worth undertaking, though inhaled triggers are also the most difficult to avoid.

Myth #7:
The steroids often given for asthma are the same medications illicitly used by athletes to build muscles.

Many parents are afraid of allergy and asthma medications classified as steroids. However, these medications are not the same as the steroids abused by athletes. While steroids used to treat asthma have their own side effects, they are an enormously valuable part of our arsenal of tools against asthma. Have your physician explain all of the real risks and real benefits before you decide. (Also refer to Chapter 13.) The very serious risk of inadequately treated asthma is important to factor in here.

Myth #8:
Any side effect from a medication means you are allergic to that medication.

If your child has had an allergic reaction to a particular medication, it is important to avoid using it again. Therefore, many children have been labeled allergic to a medication because of a side effect but not a true allergy. The commonly prescribed antibiotic amoxicillin offers a classic example. Young children sometimes develop a fine red rash while taking amoxicillin, especially when they have a viral infection. This is not an allergic reaction and is not dangerous. If your child gets a rash, run them by the doctor's office. You don't want to lose the use of an antibiotic simply because of a misunderstanding about a rash.

Liquid medications for young children cause another complication: Children sometimes develop significant reactions to the artificial coloring or flavoring, not the actual medication.

Before assuming your child is allergic to a medication, ask your doctor about this possibility.

Myth #9:
Children with asthma can't play sports.

Dozens of world-class athletes with asthma have been in the public eye, so I hope we are getting close to the end of hearing this myth. However, there is a more insidious twist to this story. Many kids themselves become convinced that they are not athletic or not good at sports because they are limited by unrecognized asthma. Children with inadequately controlled asthma often grow up sedentary without anyone making the connection, and this is a terrible shame.

Myth #10:
Hospitalizations for asthma are inevitable.

When I meet parents for the first time at their child's bedside in the hospital, I am often struck by their lack of surprise that the child has been hospitalized. While asthma can indeed sneak up on you, hospitalization should be the exception, not the rule. I repeatedly emphasize to parents of hospitalized children that the easy part is to get their child better and out of the hospital. The more important job is to analyze what was being done prior to this exacerbation and *change the plan!* Otherwise the hospital experience may be repeated.

Learning Disorders and Allergies

A question I am frequently asked concerns the relationship between allergies, hyperactivity, and learning disorders. This is a difficult issue. Certainly many children who have learning disabilities and behavioral difficulties don't have allergies. However, it is also true that poorly controlled allergies or asthma seem to contribute to the problem or exacerbate these difficulties. If sleep quality is poor, kids may be more restless and have a shortened attention span. Medications can also sometimes contribute to this problem. I learned a long time ago that the children who are very active or have a shortened attention span to begin with are the same kids who tend to develop unacceptable side effects to allergy or asthma medications. For instance, the most common side effect of antihistamines is drowsiness. Yet some children have a paradoxical reaction and become hyperactive or even agitated. This leads us to the idea that there may be some more basic connection to these two conditions, both of which seem to be increasing in frequency throughout the world. If your child has allergies or asthma and also seems to be struggling in school, talk to your child's pediatrician about possible connections between the two problems.

Could Allergies and Asthma Be Totally Prevented?

Current international guidelines refer to three categories of preventive strategies:

Primary Prevention   Strategies introduced before exposure to risk factors. The goal is to prevent allergies and asthma from occurring in the first place.

Secondary Prevention   Strategies introduced for children who are susceptible to developing allergies or asthma but do not yet have full-blown symptoms.

Tertiary Prevention   Strategies to avoid exposure to allergens and other nonspecific triggers once a child has developed full-blown allergies and asthma.

Primary prevention—stopping the allergies or asthma before a child ever reacts—would be every family's first choice solution, and indeed, this is where the future of allergy and asthma management lies. Unfortunately, at this point scientists are just beginning to unravel the details of early allergy development, with a lot of investigators focusing on the second trimester of pregnancy. The key question is whether steps taken while pregnant could lessen the likelihood of a child developing allergies or asthma in the first place.

This is tricky. You might think if a pregnant woman avoided foods known to cause food allergies, perhaps her child might be less prone to future food allergies. In fact, there is early evidence, by no means proven, that exposure to high doses of allergens by a pregnant woman, and perhaps even having immunotherapy (allergy shots) while pregnant, might result in children less likely to be allergic. And just to confuse the issue, one study suggested that low-dose allergen exposure in utero might be more likely to sensitize a baby than high-dose allergen exposure.

For many reasons, exposure to cigarette smoke during a mother's pregnancy is bad for a child, particularly those who are genetically predisposed to allergies or asthma. Poor growth of the bronchial tubes is among the side effects of exposure to nicotine. Infants of mothers who smoke are four times as likely to develop wheezing in early childhood.

Does Exposure During Infancy Make the Difference?

What about after your baby is born? Unfortunately, the jury is still out regarding early exposure to allergens. Many studies over the years have suggested that if you decrease early exposure to allergens in the first few years of life, you may decrease the likelihood of your child eventually having bad allergies or asthma. The most important cause of lifelong allergies and asthma appear to be genetic, and at this point there is nothing you can or should do about that. But working on your infant's environment may help.

For many years I have been recommending avoidance of significant environmental allergens for infants at risk of developing significant allergies. Now, I have to admit, I'm not so sure that what I've been suggesting is such a good idea after all. It is frustrating to admit how little is certain in this area.

A good example of the current confusion has to do with day care and early viral infections. Viral infections are the number one cause of wheezing in infants and toddlers, and the first asthma episode in a child's life is usually due to a viral infection. This might lead parents to think that if they could afford to keep their child out of day care and away from lots of sick children (children in day care have more early illnesses than their at-home counterparts), they might prevent their child from developing asthma. However, the story isn't that simple. We are starting to suspect that viral infections in early childhood may be important to the development of a strong immune system, and in fact it seems that children who develop stronger immunity early on are less likely to have asthma.

To complicate the picture, not all viruses seem to be created equal. You may have heard of the notorious virus named RSV (respiratory syncytial virus). RSV can be just another cold virus or, under the right circumstances, RSV can trigger bad wheezing episodes called *bronchiolitis*. This virus may make a child more prone to asthma, though the data is not yet clear.

Another related area of intense scientific interest has to do with something called *probiotics*, which can be purchased at outrageously high prices in your local health food stores. These products are purported to alter a child's normal intestinal flora, the germs that reside in your gut and help determine absorption of food and allergens into your bloodstream. While this might be a good idea, there is simply inadequate data to recommend the use of probiotics. History is filled with examples of good ideas that didn't turn out to work—or worse, made things worse. Just because something may be helpful doesn't mean it really is.

Some studies have suggested that if a woman avoids known food allergens such as cow's milk, eggs, nuts, and fish while breast-feeding, her infant may be less likely to develop eczema or atopic dermatitis. But the longest studies suggest that the benefits seem to fade over time and that after a few years their children are right back to where they started. Furthermore, sometimes these dietary manipulations may even result in babies that don't grow as well. So, all in all, I am cautious about recommending such approaches.

So what are you supposed to do with all of this information?

The bottom line is that while primary prevention of allergies and asthma may be a great idea, it is just that, a good idea whose time has not yet come. My advice is to be very wary of any fabulous claims about products purported to prevent allergies or asthma. Manufacturers, big and small, are taking advantage of the inadequacy of scientific data to separate you from your bank account. The preventive steps we know can work are fully explained in Chapter 8.

On the Increase?

In articles about allergies and asthma, the popular press frequently notes that these conditions are on the increase. While the frequency is increasing (and this is true throughout the world), it is not increasing as much as many people think. Asthma and allergies have always been common, but they frequently went unrecognized. This lack of recognition in the past was, not surprisingly, a much bigger problem in poorer areas of both the United States and developing nations. However, even in affluent suburbs, asthma frequently has gone undiagnosed or misdiagnosed; if a child mostly coughed and didn't wheeze, for example, he was generally considered to have recurrent croup, bronchitis, pneumonia, or all of the above.

Nonetheless, the true prevalence of asthma is increasing. Many investigators are naturally looking at the relationship between asthma and air pollution. Certainly asthma attacks increase whenever the air quality drops. However, asthma and allergies are increasing even in areas with fairly clean air or air cleaner than thirty years ago.

Indoor air may also be an important factor. The air in our homes, schools, and workplaces is not fresh, and of course passive smoke triggers significant coughing and wheezing. In a number of inner-city studies, proteins excreted by cockroaches are an important allergen.

But most observers do not think that air quality can fully explain the problem. There appears to be something about our modern (Western) lifestyle that may be contributing to this dramatic increase. The best advice I can give you is to keep reading the newspaper. Over the next few years, there may be some new developments that will be helpful to your family.

TAKE-HOME MESSAGES

- The symptoms of allergies and asthma sometimes masquerade as another type of health problem. If your child doesn't get better when treated for the first illness, ask your pediatrician if your child may have allergies or asthma.

- Sometimes families mistake food intolerances for food allergy. Intolerances can be quite debilitating and need to be treated, but the correct treatment is completely different.

- Allergies may worsen over time, so the earlier your child's allergic triggers are identified, the easier they will be to manage.

- Early aggressive treatment of asthma may lessen its severity as a child ages.

- Asthma should not be addressed on an attack-by-attack basis; consistent, long-term prevention and treatment is what promotes good health.

- Myths about allergies and asthma abound. When you hear or read about a new theory or treatment, check with your doctor to see if there is any validity to it.

- Scientists still have a great deal to learn about allergies and asthma. Keep asking your doctor, "What's new?"

THREE

Understanding the Causes
of Allergic Reactions

Jason is an adorable four-year-old who came to my office one day with his parents, Linda and Jeff. Normally I love to see fathers come for visits, an all-too-uncommon experience. But this time I felt the room temperature drop about 10 degrees when Jason's mom and dad came in and sat almost as far away from each other as possible. Clearly a war was going on. Christmas was a little more than a week away, and I soon heard about last year's annual trek to Jeff's parents' home in Virginia. Poor Jason had a bad asthma attack, so he spent Christmas night in a local emergency room instead of with his grandparents. As this year's trip neared, Linda was afraid for Jason, and she didn't want to travel to her in-laws' home this winter.

I don't have to tell you how important family holiday get-togethers are to almost everyone, but of course, no one wished to put little Jason through another attack like the last one. "So, Dr. Dozor, should we spend Christmas at my mom's or not?" asked Jeff. Now that is a loaded question if I ever heard one!

This family crisis demonstrates the importance of understanding the causes of allergic reactions. If we knew that Jason's problem was because of the almonds in Grandmom's pie or the beautiful fresh-cut Christmas tree he helped decorate, just think how easily this problem might be solved. Or maybe Jason and his family could make the trip, but he should skip jumping into piles of moldy leaves. Or perhaps if Jason didn't sleep in the bed normally reserved for that old dog, Rosie, all would be well.

Or maybe Jason's illness had nothing whatsoever to do with allergies. He'd been coming down with a cold when they made the trip last year—maybe his asthma was triggered by a viral infection. As Christmas was only a few days away, there wasn't time to come up with a reasonable medical answer. All I could do was make some educated guesses, help them do some family soul-searching, and book an appointment for Jason in January when we would do more in-depth analysis.

All of us—parents and physicians alike—wish we had some global answer for why kids suffer from allergies and asthma and why they are on the increase. Let me begin by explaining a little about what these scientists are exploring, and then continue with more specific information about allergies. (A full explanation of asthma can be found in Chapter 2; Part Four describes various causes and treatments.)

Allergies and Asthma on the Rise: Possible Causes

THE HYGIENE HYPOTHESIS

Recently the medical community has been puzzling over what has been referred to as the hygiene hypothesis. Several intriguing studies suggest that kids who have more frequent early childhood illnesses, usually viral infections, might actually have fewer allergies and instances of asthma when they grow older. Certainly children in day care tend to be sicker in the first few years of life—more runny noses, coughing, wheezing, ear infections, etc. Ironically, those early illnesses may play an important role in preparing the developing immune system for life. Maybe, the theory goes, the allergic response develops when you aren't busy fighting off all of those nasty viruses. In other words, maybe the increased incidence of allergies and asthma is part of the price we pay for healthier kids than in previous generations.

Immunizations

Universal immunization of children is probably the most clear-cut public health victory of the twentieth century. I am quite certain very few people would wish to go back to epidemics of polio, diphtheria, tetanus, whooping cough, measles, mumps, and rubella. Before immunizations, thousands of children in our country and throughout the world died each year of these dread diseases; many were permanently disabled. Children today receive even more vaccines than twenty years ago. Could it be that all of these immunizations alter our immune system in some unintended way, stimulating or allowing the development of allergies?

Antibiotics

After immunizations, the development of antibiotics is the next most dramatic and wonderful advance in healthcare over the last century. However, once again, aggressive treatment of illnesses may have changed the way we respond to allergens. And certainly the increased use of antibiotics has led to an increase in the number of people who are allergic to antibiotics. That concern, plus the very dramatic and frightening increase in infectious agents that are now resistant to antibiotics, are just now convincing physicians that we really need to change our prescribing practices.

So, where might all of these questions lead? No one knows for sure. If we can understand why allergies and asthma have become so frequent, maybe we can make more rational decisions about our air, our water, and our environment. Maybe if we understand the influences of early childhood, we could prevent long-term allergies and asthma.

Everyday Exposure

Children may be exposed to allergens in several different ways, each of which can trigger a variety of reactions:

1. by inhalation (ragweed, pollen)
2. by direct contact with the skin (latex, poison ivy)
3. by ingestion (nuts, shellfish)
4. By injection (penicillin, insect stings)

COMMON SYMPTOMS OF RESPIRATORY ALLERGIES

Anaphylaxis (rare!)	Headaches	Runny nose
Burning eyes	Hoarseness	Shortness of breath
Chest tightness	Impaired smell	Sneezing
Cough	Itchy nose or throat	Tingling nose
Dark circles under the eyes ("allergic shiners")	Nasal congestion	Vertigo
Difficulty swallowing	Postnasal drip	Watery, itchy, crusty, or red eyes
Difficulty sleeping	Ringing or fullness fullness in the ears	Wheezing
Fatigue		

Airborne Allergens

Parents have lots of questions: "Should we give away the cat? Should we cover the living room furniture in plastic? Vacuum daily? Keep the child off the baseball diamond in the spring? Should we raise a ruckus about the rabbit in Roger's classroom?"

Important clues to the cause of an allergy come from the "where" and "when" of the reaction. Some respiratory allergens will only tend to bother your child indoors (dust mites, animal dander, mold spores, cockroaches) since only inside will there be a significant build up of the offending substance. Some triggers are predominantly outdoors, though they certainly can fly into our homes on nice summer days when windows are open. Some, like pollens, are limited to specific seasons and specific geographic areas. Some, unfortunately, are in our environment all year. Over time many of us can figure out our seasonal or indoor allergens by paying attention to the timing of our reactions. Every spring, for instance, my hay fever is at its worst. It doesn't take a rocket scientist to figure out that the culprits are grass and tree pollens.

Here are some other examples: When I used to get down on the carpeted floor of our family room and tickle the kids, I would occasionally have a pretty good sneezing attack that was due to dust allergy. It took me a long time to figure out that my eyes water and I start sneezing whenever I am in a house with cats.

What Happens When an Allergen Hits the Airways

The nose should be the subject of an entire book. While it's terrific for holding glasses and quite adept at identifying the smell of fresh-baked cookies, the real purpose of the nose is to protect the rest of our respiratory tract. I believe it is the single most important part of our respiratory defenses. The nose is cleverly designed to catch the larger irritants before the airstream turns the corner and travels down into the bronchial tubes. Of course, if your nose is completely stuffed, as mine often is, then inhaled air must bypass the nose and travel directly from our mouths to our lungs. So, not surprisingly, people with nasal congestion are more likely to have asthmalike symptoms because irritants weren't stopped in the nose.

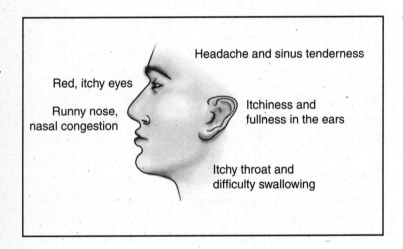

If allergens land in your upper respiratory tract (nose, mouth, and throat), the symptoms are likely to be a runny or stuffy nose, sneezing, throat-clearing due to postnasal drip, and most distinctly, itching. And everything can itch: ears, eyes, nose, and throat. I get a tickle on the roof of my mouth and have to resist the temptation to stick a pen in there and scratch it. For most of us, allergic symptoms are concentrated in these areas (nose and areas around the nose like our eyes, ears, sinuses, and throat). This cluster of symptoms is for some reason referred to as hay fever, the major problem being inflammation of the mucus membranes of the nose, or *allergic rhinitis.*

If inhaled allergens make it past the upper respiratory tract, they will land on your bronchial tubes. And if you have asthma, they can then trigger coughing, mucus production, chest tightness, wheezing, and shortness of breath.

COMMON AIRBORNE ALLERGENS

Dust

House dust is very complex, made up of breakdown materials from all kinds of things in your home, such as stuffing material, furniture, food, and fibers. All of those ingredients may irritate the respiratory tract of people with allergies and asthma, but by far the most important ingredient appears to be dust mites, those tiny little creatures that live and die in our dust.

Pollens

Weeds, such as ragweed, sagebrush, tumbleweed, redroot pigweed, English plaintain, careless weed, spiny amaranth, or burning bush. Grasses, such as timothy, Bermuda, redtop, rye, orchard, sweet vernal, or bluegrass. Trees, such as elm, oak, maple, birch, ash, pecan, poplar, cottonwood.

Mold Spores

Indoor molds (mildew) will grow anywhere in the house that is both warm and damp, so bathrooms, showers, and basements are favorite locations. Some types of mold are *Aspergillus, Penicillium, Mucor,* and *Rhizopus.*

Outdoor molds grow in soil and in wet leaves, and

they are blown far distances on windy days. Common mold species in North America include *Alternaria, Hormodendrum,* and *Claudosporium.*

Animal Dander

Cats, dogs, birds, and all kinds of furry friends.

Cockroaches

These ubiquitous creatures are an indoor allergen.

Nonspecific Irritants

Our air is filled with all kinds of irritants, including cigarette smoke, pollutants, and fumes. Although strictly speaking these do not trigger an IgE-mediated allergic reaction, people with allergies seem to be bothered much more by these kinds of irritants than people without allergies.

Skin or Direct Contact Allergens

COMMON SYMPTOMS OF SKIN ALLERGIES

Blisters	Sandpaper skin
Dry patches	Skin thickening
Infected rashes	Swelling
Itchiness	Welts (hives)
Redness	

Allergic reactions to substances that touch our skin are very common. They can be highly uncomfortable, but usually are not too serious. The body's response may range from a little itching and puffiness to blistering, or a full-scale case of hives.

Hives, or *urticaria,* are very common, and many times we never do figure out what triggers them. In general, if hives are localized then they are probably set off by direct contact to that area. However, if hives develop and spread throughout the body, the trigger or allergen somehow got into the bloodstream. Foods and medications sometimes trigger generalized hives.

Another common and uncomfortable skin reaction is *eczema,* a term used to describe a variety of skin conditions that manifest themselves as dryness, itching, inflammation, and thickening of the skin. The symptoms may come and go. These kinds of skin rashes may not be allergic in nature (not due to an IgE-mediated reaction to a foreign protein), but rather an irritation of the skin through other mechanisms. Your skin has all kinds of amazing ways to fend off the outside world, or as they say, keep the outside out and the inside in. And many times the actual trigger, whether it was a true allergen or just some kind of nonspecific irritant, remains unrecognized.

Atopic dermatitis refers to a subtype of eczema that appears to be predominantly allergic in nature. It is often difficult to control. Atopic dermatitis tends to be most pronounced in children, and they almost always show other signs of being allergic or atopic, such as hives, hay fever, or asthma. Infants and children with atopic dermatitis seem to have decreased skin oil production and love to scratch even the tiniest patch.

Here are some of the common causes of skin allergies:

PLANTS

Almost half of all people are allergic to poison ivy, sumac, and oak. An oily resin on the plants sets off the reaction, and for those who are very allergic, an amazingly tiny amount of that stuff can trigger a pretty nasty rash. If your child is allergic to these plants, she will not only react after direct contact, but sometimes from touching clothing or pets that have been exposed. Keep in mind that you usually have to be exposed repeatedly before your body develops an allergic reaction. Many parents find it pretty confusing when their child had no problem in the past and then suddenly they do.

One common misunderstanding is that scratching or breaking the blisters will cause the rash to spread. None of the irritating resin, called urushiol, is in the blisters so this isn't possible. However, your child can certainly make things a lot worse by scratching and irritating the rash.

There are other plants that cause allergic reactions, some of which still remain unnamed. But tulips, daisies, chrysanthemums, sagebrush, and heliotrope, which grow in the southwest deserts, are well-known triggers. All of these plants can cause rashes if you brush up against them, so try to convince kids to wear long pants and socks while scampering around in the desert!

COSMETICS

Allergic reactions to cosmetics are pretty rare when you consider how many chemicals are in these products. Of course, unlike the manufacturers of insecticides and antifreeze, cosmetic companies go to a great deal of effort to try and make sure these are safe, which in the past was not a good deal for bunny rabbits and other animals that have been used in the testing. But certainly such items as eye makeup, lipstick, perfume, hair dye, etc. can all trigger allergic reactions. If your adolescent daughter starts experimenting with makeup and starts sporting apple-red cheeks that are not from blush, the cosmetics may be the cause.

I remember one family trip out to Arizona and New Mexico, when my wife decided to shower with fancy and heavily perfumed soap at a beautiful bed and breakfast. She came out of the shower red and swollen from top to bottom.

Remember, too, that your child need not actually be the one using the perfume to have a reaction. If she comes into contact with these chemicals while you're giving her a good hug before heading out to the movies or if the teacher puts on a goodly dose in the morning, your child may react.

CHEMICALS

All kinds of metals and other chemicals have been known to cause allergic reactions. Like all allergens, low-level exposure over many years generally leads to the development of a reaction. Even then the reactions sometimes don't appear until one to two days after contact and can last for days or weeks. The time delay aspect of the reaction means that it can be very tricky to figure out the root cause.

Formaldehyde is a particularly common trigger, since it is found in a long list of places in our homes. This nasty stuff can escape as an odorless gas from such things as wallboard, insulation, furniture, rugs, clothing (particularly permanent-press), and even car exhaust. So the next time you notice a burning sensation in your eyes or nose for no apparent reason, that could easily be a reaction to this almost ubiquitous chemical.

Alas, the list of chemicals in our environment grows daily. Some cause itchy rashes, and some, such as film developing chemicals and rubber, can cause significant hives and even serious generalized reactions. Many household products such as antifreeze and insecticides are notorious for creating problems.

METALS

Nickel is the metal most likely to cause a reaction, and it is often found in inexpensive earrings or other jewelry. If your child develops a rash from the snap on a pair of jeans or from any rivets on clothing, think nickel allergy.

Lots of other metals have also been known to trigger reactions, such as mercury, chrome, and beryllium. These exposures tend to be work related, and it would be unlikely for a child to be exposed to these substances.

LATEX

A very important allergic trigger is latex. Latex has become ubiquitous in many environments, particularly in the world of healthcare. (I doubt there is a single nurse or physician who hasn't watched the explosion in the use of latex gloves during the last twenty years and thought to themselves, "Gee, I sure wish I made these gloves.")

I care for one child with a known latex allergy whose mother wisely brings a latex-free stethoscope to my office. Without a stethoscope where would I be?

A child who has had multiple surgical procedures can develop a latex allergy, and this often goes unrecognized. If your belly is opened for some reason (never a good idea if you can avoid it), your intestines can be exposed to significant amounts of the latex during surgery. Some children have had life-threatening and even fatal reactions after repeated exposures to latex under these circumstances. Children born with certain conditions, such as spina bifida, are at particularly high risk for these reactions. And these kids often require lots of contact with doctors and hospitals. Some hospitals, particularly children's hospitals, have been able to set up completely latex-free operating rooms. This could be life saving. In Chapter 18, you'll find more information on latex.

COMMON CAUSES OF SKIN ALLERGIES

Common:	Less common:
Plants	
poison ivy, oak, and sumac	heliotrope, chrysanthemums sagebrush, wormwood, tulips, daisies
Cosmetics	
Eye makeup and eye shadow	Nail polishes
Hair products	Antiperspirants
Lipstick	Perfumes
Chemicals	
Latex	Chlorine
Formaldehyde	Phenols
Alcohols	
Metals	
Nickel	Mercury
Chrome	Beryllium
Drugs	
Local anesthetics, e.g., Novocaine	Neomycin
Penicillin	Streptomycin
Sulfa	

Insect Allergies

If your child is stung or bitten by an insect, comfort them, tell them their pain won't last long, and the redness and itching should fade in a couple of hours. However, the fear and anxiety both children and parents develop about insects may last a lifetime, because some people develop true allergic reactions. They may be mild and involve only local swelling and redness at the bite. Rarely, insect bites trigger massive allergic reactions, which, if not treated, can be very serious and even life-threatening. About fifty deaths each year in the United States can be attributed to insect sting allergy.

INSECTS THAT CAUSE ALLERGIC REACTIONS

Serious Reactions	Mild Reactions
Bumble bees	Mosquitoes
Honey bees	Spiders
Yellow jackets	Ticks
Wasps	Biting flies
Hornets	Fire ants

People are not actually allergic to the insect, but to some of the proteins in the venom, triggering what is known as a hypersensitivity reaction. Interestingly, the chemicals that cause nasty local pain and irritation are not the same ones that trigger true allergic reactions. Some insects, such as mosquitoes, spiders, ticks, or biting flies, are associated with mild reactions, while others, including bees, yellow jackets, wasps, hornets, and fire ants, have been known to cause very serious reactions.

Some allergic reactions to an insect sting begin almost immediately, and these early reactions are potentially the most serious. Local reactions, such as pain and mild swelling, may immediately occur. Then within about ten to twenty minutes, more generalized symptoms, that originate from other parts of the body such as hives, wheezing, or shortness of breath, let you know that the allergic reaction is becoming generalized and not limited to just the location of the sting or bite.

Key Point: *If you suspect that your child is developing a more generalized reaction, this is a true medical emergency and she needs to be taken to the emergency room as soon as possible.*

COMMON SYMPTOMS OF INSECT STING ALLERGY

Abdominal cramps	Itchy eyes
Bluish color around the lips and mouth	Nausea
Chest tightness	Sense of confusion
Collapse	Shock
Constricted throat	Slurred speech
Coughing	Swelling extending far from the bite
Difficulty breathing	Vomiting
Dizziness	

If you or your child ever has any of these systemic symptoms, it is very important that you see an allergist and that you are prepared for any future stings. After one serious reaction, the majority of people will have a serious reaction again the next time they are stung.

Drug Allergies

Like other allergies, severe allergic reactions to medications or other drugs only occur after repeated exposure, not the first time a medicine is introduced.

Penicillin allergy is the most commonly reported drug allergy. Actually, plain penicillin isn't prescribed that often anymore, and therefore most allergic reactions are to antibiotics in the same chemical category, such as ampicillin, amoxicillin, Augmentin, and all of the antibiotics known as cephalosporins. These compounds share some of their structure but other areas are quite different. So the specific IgE your child has produced after previous exposure to one drug in this group may not actually bind to a new drug. This is quite fortunate, because I am always meeting patients who are labeled with a penicillin allergy but tolerate related antibiotics without difficulty.

It is also true that some children are labeled allergic to penicillin who really aren't. That is because children occasionally develop a fine red non-itchy rash while taking either of two common antibiotics, amoxicillin or ampicillin. This rash appears to occur most often when kids are actually ill with a viral infection. It is very important to have your pediatrician or family doctor take a look at this rash, since this is not a sign of true allergy and your children do not need to be deprived of these valuable medications.

To complicate the situation, children sometimes appear to be having an allergic reaction to certain medications but actually are reacting to the flavorings or coloring compounds used in many preparations. Certain food colorings are notorious for causing reactions and are sometimes found in liquid medications.

Antibiotics derived from sulfa, such as Gantrisen, Bactrim, or Septra, are known for their tendency to trigger allergic reactions. So are some of the common medications used to treat seizures.

More and more X-ray studies these days, particularly CAT scans and MRI scans, are done with injection of special dyes designed to enhance the value of these important tests. A wide variety of these agents have been developed for specific tests, and many have been reported to trigger allergic reactions, though rarely in children. In fact, an increasing number of radiologists are routinely insisting that children with asthma be pretreated with prednisone or other corticosteroids before the injection.

Some people, usually adults, develop hives or asthma when taking aspirin. This is not true allergy but a unique reaction to aspirin and the other pain relievers related to asthma.

COMMON SYMPTOMS OF DRUG ALLERGIES

Coughing	Joint pains
Fevers	Skin rashes
Hives	Sneezing
Itching	Wheezing

The most common symptoms of drug allergies are hives or similar rashes that usually appear within an hour. Rarely, allergic reactions will appear one to three days afterward and that can confuse the issue. Also, after an allergic reaction to an antibiotic, hives may wax and wane for a few weeks after the last dose was actually taken.

Penicillin and related drugs are also known to cause a prolonged allergic reaction called *serum sickness*. In this situation, fevers, swollen glands, joint pains, and rashes may develop a few weeks after taking the medication.

Essentially any drug can trigger an allergic reaction, but amazingly, most allergic reactions are triggered by a relatively small list of medications, and allergic reactions to drugs not on this list are fairly uncommon.

DRUGS THAT COMMONLY CAUSE ALLERGIC REACTIONS

Anticonvulsants, e.g., Dilantin	Insulin
Amoxicillin	Local anesthetics, e.g., Novocaine
Ampicillin	Penicillin
Augmentin	Phenobarbital (barbiturates)
Cephalosporins	Sulfa drugs
	Tetracycline

Food Allergies

Food allergies may be very recognizable when a reaction occurs right after eating the offending food. Unfortunately, pinning down food allergies is sometimes much trickier. Our modern diet is very complex, including many known and unknown ingredients that may cause allergic reactions. Your child's reactions to certain foods may be quite variable, occurring only with certain quantities or frequency of ingestion. Cooking methods and times may change the allergic nature of a food, too. We will review the diagnostic tests in a later chapter, but proving food allergies can be very tough.

Overwhelming allergic reactions to foods (anaphylaxis) such as nuts or shellfish unfortunately can occur to any child. This is a nightmare and will be discussed in more detail in a later chapter.

COMMON SYMPTOMS OF FOOD ALLERGIES

Abdominal pains	Nasal congestion
Cramps	Nausea or vomiting
Diarrhea	Runny nose
Eczema	Swelling of the eyes, lips, face, or tongue
Hives	

Food allergies, however, are perhaps the most confusing of the types of allergic reactions. Specific foods may trigger terrible symptoms, but this may not be due to a true allergic reaction, in the sense of an IgE-mediated response as we have previously discussed. For instance, as discussed in Chapter 2, many people develop stomachaches and diarrhea after drinking cow's milk due to lactase deficiency. Some people gradually develop lactase deficiency as they grow older, and this can be easily diagnosed. One key difference between milk intolerance due to lactase deficiency and true milk allergy is that you may still be able to tolerate yogurt, sour cream, or even some cheeses, because most of the lactose is already broken down.

Food intolerances may not be as potentially serious as true allergy, but they certainly can be frightening. My brother, Barry, was the first person I knew who regularly developed "Chinese Restaurant Syndrome." This is an uncommon reaction to MSG (monosodium glutamate), a very popular flavor enhancer. It used to scare the heck out of him. Gradually he would develop this warm feeling at the back of his neck, then sweating and dizziness, and eventually almost faint. Not allergic but not very nice.

COMMON FOOD ALLERGENS

Beans	Milk
Berries	Nuts
Chocolate	Shellfish
Corn	Soy
Eggs	Wheat
Food thickeners (gum arabic)	

To summarize, your child might develop an allergic reaction to just about anything, but fortunately, most of the time these reactions are not too severe. Since severe and even life-threatening reactions can and do occur, it is very important to recognize when an allergic reaction is taking place. For example, the very worst drug allergies I have seen have been in children who continued taking the medication for many days after symptoms of allergy began. It can be very tricky to identify the true cause of an allergic reaction since there are so many different potential triggers, and the time course of reactions can be so variable. If your child is having symptoms suggestive of an allergic reaction, don't jump to conclusions. Rather, analyze the situation carefully. Failure to recognize a true allergen can have very serious and long-term consequences.

TAKE-HOME MESSAGES

- Allergic reactions are very common, but fortunately, usually mild.

- Not all skin rashes or other symptoms are due to true allergic reactions, and it is important to distinguish between intolerances or side effects and true allergy.

- If your child is having symptoms that you think might be allergic, think about possible triggers—that is, foreign substances landing on that part of the body.

- Respiratory symptoms (sneezing, coughing, and wheezing) are most likely due to reactions to airborne allergens, not food allergies.

- Hives and rashes are most commonly from direct skin contact, though an ingested or injected allergen may cause a systemic or generalized reaction.

- If your child seems to be developing more generalized symptoms coming from more than one part of their body, this could be very serious. He or she requires immediate medical attention.

PART TWO:

IN SEARCH OF A SOLUTION

FOUR

Consulting the Doctor: Pediatrician, Family Physician, or Specialist?

Caroline is a very bright three-year-old who has seen more than her fair share of doctors. Caroline has asthma, and she has been to her pediatrician's office four times this winter with wheezing; each time she needed urgent care. As a result, she saw a different partner in her doctor's group each visit. She also was seen by her mother's dermatologist when her eczema flared out of control, and she had two visits to an ear, nose, and throat specialist because of drainage from her ears. But with all of that "crisis management," no one was looking at the big picture—attempting to organize an overall management plan. Without an organized approach, Caroline was doomed to spend the rest of the winter bouncing from crisis to crisis.

Start with Your Pediatrician or Family Physician

If your child is having symptoms that suggest either allergies or asthma, your first stop should be with your primary care provider. A primary care provider is someone who specializes in taking care of the whole child, and that can be a very important and useful viewpoint. This person could be a pediatrician, family physician, or nurse practitioner. It is estimated that primary care providers can manage 30 to 50 percent of children with allergies and asthma, and when possible, this is ideal. It's easier for the family, and it saves the additional time and expense of visiting a specialist.

In addition, if your pediatrician or family doctor is personable, enthusiastic, and knows your child, those are really important skills to bring to the job. Those qualifications are sometimes more important than specialized training.

Most people hope to lump allergy or asthma care into their child's annual well-child checkup. While some issues can be resolved on this occasion, those yearly visits are designed to survey all kinds of different issues (growth, immunizations, general health of the child), not to focus on one or two specific problems. If your child is having significant allergies or asthma, I urge you to make a separate appointment with your primary care provider designed just to discuss these issues. And it will help if it is possible to leave your other children at home so you can focus solely on the issues pertaining to the child whose health is being scrutinized.

Key Point: *In this book I will usually refer to healthcare providers as doctors or physicians. This is not to slight nurse practitioners who are often just as competent as any physician and sometimes have more time to be thorough. In today's healthcare environment, the time available to spend helping you and your child is critical to successfully handling the problem.*

The Goals of Allergy and Asthma Management

My goals for any patient are really quite simple: I want your children to be able to do anything they want, participate fully in all activities, and not feel limited by these conditions. I don't want your children's symptoms to affect their lifestyle. In the process, I want to use the least amount of medication possible to achieve those goals, and I don't want any side effects from the medications.

Take note that I didn't say "no symptoms." It is important to realize that all humans sneeze, cough, and develop rashes on occasion. That's okay.

When are these reactions not okay? They are not okay when symptoms are affecting your child to the point that she is more than a little uncomfortable or her life is disrupted by the symptoms. If your child wakes in the middle of the night coughing, that is not okay. If your child's nose is so stuffy she can't breathe through it and can't taste food, that's not okay. If she has a low-level cough or other symptoms almost every day, even between acute respiratory illnesses, that's not okay. If your child ends up in the emergency room, in the hospital, missing a lot of school, sitting out parts of soccer games, or unable to complete the mile run at school, that's not acceptable.

By the same token, the level of medication must be acceptable. If your child is up all night or falling asleep during the day because of allergy medicines, that's not okay. If she is feeling jittery for hours after using an inhaler, that's not okay. If she requires more than very occasional courses of oral prednisone (corticosteroids), that's not okay.

SUGGESTED GOALS FOR ALLERGY
AND ASTHMA CARE

- Symptoms should not affect your child's lifestyle.
- Your child should be able to participate in all activities, including sports.
- There should be no hospitalization and no emergency room visits.
- Your child should not miss a lot of school.
- There should be no side effects from the medications.
- Your child should be completely well in between colds or other illnesses.
- Your child's symptoms should not disrupt sleep.
- The least amount of medicine possible should be used to achieve all of the above.

Ultimately only you and your child can decide whether the regimen you are using is meeting your needs.

Prior to the Appointment with Your Doctor

Think through the purpose of the appointment. What are your child's symptoms? When and where do they occur? If your child is currently on medications, write down the exact dosage or take the containers with you. Make a note of what your goals are for the appointment: What can't your child do right now that you would like her to be able to do? By preparing in advance, you will keep from forgetting important questions. If the doctor is running late or your child is restless, a list of things to discuss with the doctor will help keep you from feeling frazzled.

Here is a list of common and important questions:

QUESTIONS TO ASK YOUR DOCTOR

- Does my child have allergies or asthma?
- Could there be anything else going on besides allergies and asthma?
- If my child does have allergies, what are his triggers?
- Should my child have allergy testing?
- Should my child see a specialist, and if so, should it be an allergist or pulmonologist?
- What else besides allergies might trigger my child's asthma?
- How can I prevent or limit my child's exposure to allergens?
- Should my child be given allergy shots?
- How often should I see you?
- Does my child need medication all of the time or just when he is symptomatic?
- What side effects of the medications should I watch for?
- Do I need to worry about any side effects?
- Is there a safer way to manage my child?
- If my child is being treated intermittently, how do I decide when to start and when to stop the medications?
- What do I do if the prescribed medications are not working adequately or have unacceptable side effects?
- Whom should I call for refills?
- Whom should I call in an emergency?

The Important Role of the Parent

As a parent, you are the most important member of the diagnostic team, as the descriptions of symptoms and the past medical history of the child are key elements. When visiting a specialist, it is better if both parents can be there at least the first time. Parents often have slightly different takes on the situation.

I hope this doesn't sound too sexist, but I'm often disappointed when only Dad brings a child in for that first visit. There are, of course, many exceptions, but dads often seem a lot hazier about details. In most families, mothers are primarily responsible for dealing with health issues, and they seem to have the history burned into their brains forever. Visits with just Dad are quicker, but often less complete.

Recently I've noticed a number of dads who immediately let me know that they would like to get Mom on the phone at work so I can take a history from her. When this first happened, I was a little put off, since taking a history is an art best done up close and personal. Now I've gotten used to it and have learned to make the best of it.

Regardless of whether both parents can make it, the better prepared you are, the more useful a doctor's visit will be. If you are taking your child to someone new to you, remember that she will want to go over your child's past medical history in considerable detail. Try to remember any relevant points; even things you don't think are important. Family history is important but usually less so than the personal history of the child in question. (Chapter 5 describes what kind of information a doctor is looking for when he takes a patient's history.)

Making an Assessment

I suspect pediatricians are often unaware when parents are not satisfied. As a parent, your obligation is to speak up. Let the doctor know that you would like your child to be doing better. While a specialist may be needed for more complex allergies or asthma, the solution for some children may be as simple as switching daily allergy medicines. You need to consider the following:

- Am I confident that my primary care provider has the diagnosis pinned down?
- What are the goals of any medical regimen suggested for my child?
- Are the medications my child is taking meeting our needs?

And ultimately, you'll want to ask yourself this question:

- Am I happy with how things are going?

In my experience, the biggest mistake parents make is to settle before their child's symptoms are controlled satisfactorily.

What If Your Primary Care Provider Doesn't Have Things Under Control?

You're in charge of your child's health. If you have consulted your primary care provider and feel that your goals are not being met, then it is time to see a specialist.

This does not necessarily mean the specialist should completely take over care of your child's allergies or asthma. It is usually easier, faster, and less expensive to see the specialist for just a few visits and then let your primary care provider take over from there. Some specialized diagnostic testing, additional information from someone who knows all about the field, or someone to help you evaluate the pros and cons of various treatments may be possible in a visit or two. Specialists are often harder to reach and have more limited office hours. Of course, if your child has moderate or severe allergies or asthma, an allergy or asthma specialist should perhaps be more involved.

WHEN TO REQUEST A SPECIALIST
- When the diagnosis is uncertain.
- When your primary care provider is unable to control your child's symptoms.
- When your child's asthma or allergies are moderate or severe.
- When you feel you need additional information.

ALLERGIST OR PULMONOLOGIST?

If you reach the stage when you need a specialist, you may be referred to either an allergist or a pulmonologist. While the background and education of a physician is much less important than the individual personal skills and abilities of the physician, it may be helpful to understand the distinctions between these specialties.

Allergists are experts in determining the causes of allergic reactions, performing allergy tests, advising you on what environmental controls can be put into place to prevent allergies, and in the use of immunotherapy (allergy shots). They have been around much longer than pediatric pulmonologists, and are often an excellent option.

Pediatric pulmonology is a relatively new field, and pulmonologists are most often found at large academic medical centers or children's hospitals. They are diagnosticians and usually manage children with much rarer respiratory illnesses. They are best prepared to explain why a child is coughing for months on end and why the prescribed medications aren't working adequately, and to determine what may be missed in a child who continues to suffer bothersome symptoms. They also tend to be experts in interpreting a variety of tests that measure lung function—so-called pulmonary function tests—which can be very useful.

ALLERGIST OR PULMONOLOGIST?

Allergist	Pulmonologist
Specialist in the diagnosis and treatment of allergic diseases and asthma	Specialist in the diagnosis and treatment of all respiratory tract illness, including asthma
Specialized skills:	**Specialized skills:**
Allergy testing	Interpretation of pulmonary function tests
Environmental controls	Bronchoscopy and other diagnostic tests
Immunotherapy	Diagnosis and management of patients with rare respiratory illnesses

Some kids benefit from having *both* an allergist and a pulmonologist. They are not mutually exclusive. However, most kids really don't need both since either should be expert at prescribing medications and safely controlling your child's symptoms.

Before becoming specialists, most doctors will have trained as either a pediatrician or an internist. If given the choice, bring your child to a specialist with pediatric credentials. There may be a significant difference in style.

Bring Relevant Health Records

If you are taking your child to a specialist for the first time, it is important to bring copies of medical records. Results of any previous allergy tests or pulmonary function tests can save a lot of time. If your child ever had any X-rays, try to bring copies of the actual films, not just reports. (A picture is worth a thousand words.) If your child has seen any other specialists, don't be afraid to tell the new doctor and bring copies of their reports to your primary care providers. I am always surprised when parents tell me their child had an abnormal chest X-ray recently but didn't think to bring it.

Don't assume your primary care provider has sent records when you requested them. And if they were sent, don't assume they made it from the mail and into the chart. The safest way, if possible, is to bring them with you.

At the Appointment

Many parents feel rushed during an office visit, either by the physician or their own schedule. You probably waited a long time for that appointment, so make it worthwhile. Work from your list of questions and make certain that everything is answered. (The complete diagnostic process is described in Chapter 5.)

Make certain that the doctor has clearly outlined—and you clearly understand—your plan. Many parents leave a doctor's office confused, and if your child's symptoms are intermittent or seasonal, it could be months before you have to put the plan into action. If the doctor does not write down the plan, take notes. Be sure you understand it completely.

The plan should not be to just "call the doctor" when your child is coughing or wheezing. A good doctor will encourage you to call if you are concerned, but also provide you with a systematic method for using medications properly. When symptoms are well managed, you should feel like you can control them most of the time.

The Importance of Periodic Allergy or Asthma Checkups

Remember, too, that children are always changing and their allergy and asthma therapy will have to change with them. I have never yet met a child for whom one medical regimen remained optimal for many years. And that doesn't necessarily mean they will need newer or more medicine. Sometimes they actually need less. If your children are completely asymptomatic, perhaps they are taking too much medicine. Plus, newer medications and options are always becoming available. Periodic review of your child's health plan is important.

All national and international allergy and asthma guidelines recommend periodic follow-up visits separate from routine healthcare maintenance visits. The frequency of these visits will vary depending on how your child is doing, but in my opinion, they should be at least once a year. In my own practice, I insist on every six months, whether parents feel they need it or not. I know that everyone's life is busy, and that every six months might be difficult. But I find that after longer intervals, memory fades: Which child had an ear infection over February vacation? Whose symptoms always start with coughing? How did that illness last September really start? Has your child responded adequately? What worked and what didn't? At every visit to your primary care provider, don't leave without discussing when the next appointment should be scheduled.

STEPS TO SUCCESSFUL ALLERGY
AND ASTHMA CONTROL

STEP #1:   Assess the goals you have for your
           child and if the regimen you are using
           is meeting your needs.

STEP #2:   Plan on visits just to discuss your child's
           allergies and asthma—separate from
           routine checkups.

STEP #3:   Speak up. Don't settle for less than
           optimal control. Have written questions
           and make sure you get answers that you
           understand before you leave.

STEP #4:   Don't leave the office without a written
           action plan.

STEP #5:   Insist on regularly scheduled follow-up
           visits, even if your child is well.

THE POINT OF THE VISIT

Every physician will make different recommendations, and
while it may seem confusing at first, follow their guidelines.
Only after you can report back about what works or what
doesn't work can your doctor adjust the medications to find
the right one or the right combination that will help your
child.

The key to success is to be clear about what your goals are
for the treatment of your child's allergies and asthma and
keep working at it to find the right doctors and the right medical regimen to meet your needs.

TAKE-HOME MESSAGES

- Clarify the goals you have for the care of your child's asthma and allergies.
- If possible, work with your primary care provider to meet those goals.
- If your primary care provider has not been able to control your child's symptoms, insist on a referral to a specialist.
- Prepare for doctor's visits with details about past medical history and environmental history, as well as results of any previous testing.
- Expect your child's needs to change over time.
- Plan on periodic scheduled visits devoted just to these problems.
- Don't leave the doctor's office without a written plan.
- Write down any questions you might have before your appointment.
- Ask your physicians to use the least amount of medicine necessary.

FIVE

Reaching a Diagnosis

Parents often ask, "Can't my doctor make a diagnosis of allergies or asthma without putting my child through all those tests?"

The only answer I can give is, "Sometimes." Sometimes the diagnosis is very clear. Other times tests really are necessary to clarify the diagnosis. Both parents and children should be told the tests really aren't that bad.

I'll never forget a father named Joe Weiker. (I'll mention this family and their experiences with dog allergies in a later chapter devoted to pet allergies). Joe firmly believed that his son had to have a dog. Harold sneezed, coughed, and wheezed every time he was around a dog, but it took many episodes to convince Dad of the obvious.

Primary care physicians know a very important rule of medicine, a rule, incidentally, that I frequently repeat to medical students and young physicians: *Common illnesses are a lot more common than uncommon ones.*

Even if your child's symptoms are a bit unusual, that does not necessarily mean there is something seriously wrong. Remember the corollary to the first rule: *Uncommon presentations of common illnesses are more common than uncommon illnesses.*

Anxious parents and young physicians often start by searching for unusual conditions. This is understandable when your child's symptoms either do not seem to be responding to any medications prescribed or are not resolving. However, physicians who order a battery of untargeted tests may be overdoing it. While you certainly don't want anything to be missed, your child shouldn't have to be put through any diagnostic procedures or X-rays. While these tests may be completed by a specialist, much of the process can be handled by your primary care provider. As indicated in Chapter 4, you may be able to achieve satisfactory results without ever having to consult a specialist.

The Diagnostic Process

An allergy or pulmonary evaluation is a multistep process, starting with a complete history and physical examination. Further diagnostic tests are only appropriate if the diagnosis is still uncertain.

STEP 1: COMPLETE HISTORY

While a physical exam is very important and diagnostic tests may be necessary, the answer usually lies in a family's story.

ELEMENTS OF A COMPLETE HISTORY
- Chief complaint/history of present illness
- Past medical history
- Allergy history
- Environmental history
- Dietary history
- Family history
- Social history

Chief Complaint/History of Present Illness

The initial challenge is to identify the primary problem and never lose sight of it, so the first part of the history focuses on the main reason for the visit. This may seem simple, but in fact a good diagnostician will ask a series of questions designed to rule out other causes for your child's symptoms besides allergies and asthma.

She may ask questions such as the following: How long has your child been coughing, sneezing, or itching? How did it start? Are the symptoms worse at night or during the day? Do they occur while your child is asleep? Are they worse in the morning? Indoors? Outdoors? Worsened with exercise? What seems to make them better or worse? Has any prescription or over-the-counter remedy helped? What is the nature of the symptoms? If the problem is coughing, is the cough wet, dry, barky, hacky, nonstop, spasmodic, getting worse, getting better?

When allergies are suspected, your physician may ask you to recall the specific timing of the symptoms and the temporal relationship of the symptoms to possible exposures, such as foods, seasonal allergens, environments, pets, etc. Recalling this information can be quite tricky and is sometimes misleading. There are often far too many potential triggers to easily pinpoint them. Parents frequently relate their child's current problem to previous difficulties that were incorrectly diagnosed, and this may lead to a repeat of the same mistake.

This reminds me of Mrs. McDonald, who was convinced that her two-year-old daughter, Sarah, should avoid all milk products. When Sarah was about eight weeks old, she was having terrible cramps that seemed to resolve after she was switched from her usual baby formula to a soy-based formula. In fact, Sarah's colic was not due to a cow's milk allergy, and her mom really didn't have to limit her daughter's diet at all.

Another common example has to do with penicillin allergy. A child may present with hives and itching while taking an antibiotic, and everyone assumes she is allergic to that particular medication. But her rash might not have been due to an allergic reaction, or her hives could have been an allergic reaction to something else, just coincidental to the use of the antibiotics. A good diagnostician will always strive to distinguish between what has actually been observed from what has been assumed.

Past Medical History

This is where your primary care physician has a great advantage over a doctor you are seeing for the first time. Unfortunately, more and more patients are forced to switch their primary care provider when their employer decides to switch health plans. This is too bad, because the past medical history is a treasure trove of helpful information, and it is often very difficult to recollect. The older the child and the more siblings he has, the more difficult it is for parents to remember what actually happened. If your primary care physician was involved in past episodes, the chart can be an invaluable resource. Again, having both parents come to the appointment increases the odds of remembering details.

Allergy History

The more you are able to remember about your child's symptoms and her whereabouts at the time of a reaction, the more clues the doctor will have. Your physician must separate out what is known from what is just assumed. You may think your child is allergic to your brother's cat, when actually it may be the mold in his basement.

Environmental History

When your doctor takes an "environmental history," it means she is looking for elements in the home environment that might contribute to allergies or asthma. Below is a brief list of important questions your doctor will ask at your appointment. Before your doctor's visit, think if there are any environmental questions you may have.

ENVIRONMENTAL HISTORY

- Any cigarette smoke in the home?
- What kind of heat do you have?
- Do you have central air-conditioning?
- If you have either air-conditioning or forced-hot-air heat, are there filters?
- How often are filters changed or cleaned?
- If forced air, where is the furnace?
- Does it ever smell musty or like mildew?
- Do you commonly use humidifiers or dehumidifiers?
- Which rooms have wall-to-wall carpeting?
- What kinds of window treatments are in your child's room?
- Have you made any attempts at reducing dust in your child's room?
- Are there any sources of pollution near your home that concern you?
- Do you have a lot of plants?
- Do you have pets? Where do they roam?
- Do you have concerns about cockroaches or other infestations?

Dietary History

Depending on your child's problem, a dietary history may be important. (Pinning down food allergies can be quite tricky and worthy of a whole chapter, see Chapter 6.)

Family History

Unfortunately, a history of allergies and asthma in the family isn't usually that helpful. In the last twenty years, these conditions have become so common that you can almost always find a family history of the conditions if you dig far enough. That said, we do find that having a mother or siblings with allergies or asthma definitely increases the chance of a child being affected; Dad doesn't seem to count quite as much, and more distant relatives with allergies or asthma are too common to be significant.

Occasionally I find parents who insist that there is no family history of allergies or asthma, and this is a very helpful piece of information, or what is known as a *pertinent negative*. A negative family history is so uncommon nowadays that the possibility is much greater that your child's symptoms are due to something else.

Social History

It is often helpful to understand a little about a child's daily activities. Where do they go to school? How are they doing academically and socially? What after-school and weekend activities are they involved with? Parents are always surprised when questions turn to the child's social situation and emotional adjustment. Emotional stress clearly plays a role, at least in exacerbating the symptoms or heightening the perception of symptoms. The age of a child can also make a big difference. Young adolescents, for instance, are often very tuned in to the slightest change in how they feel. While an eight-year-old or a seventeen-year-old might not be aware of fairly severe wheezing, a twelve-year-old may complain of terrible chest pains and shortness of breath even with a very mild degree of bronchospasm. Sometimes this results in a significant discrepancy between the child's description of the problem and that of the parents. Often parents, teachers, and athletic coaches will wonder if there is anything going on at all, particularly when a child has chronic complaints that don't seem to be confirmed by physical examination. However, this is an important rule I always follow: *When in doubt, believe the child.*

If a youngster feels something is going on, they are almost always right. The severity of the problem may be objectively less (or more) than would be suggested by the history, but with very rare exceptions they are not making things up. Shortness of breath or chest pains with exercise are common complaints parents may dismiss. In my experience, these symptoms are almost always real and should not be pooh-poohed.

Unfortunately, some doctors may brush off children's complaints too quickly. Sometimes parents need to step in to be certain the doctor listens to a child's concerns and treats them seriously. Ideally, a physician will listen carefully and reassure the child that his problems, while real, are easily controllable, sometimes even without drugs.

One last point: The adequacy of the history does not necessarily correlate with the time spent obtaining it. Some healthcare providers are able to collect the necessary information more quickly than others, particularly if the old chart is well documented.

STEP 2: PHYSICAL EXAMINATION

Unbeknownst to parent or child, an experienced clinician begins the physical examination at the time he or she first enters the room. Much can be learned from careful observation of such things as a patient's growth and development, skin and facial coloration, and the depth, rate, and work associated with breathing.

During an exam, I always ask myself: "What is the likelihood that anything else is going on, *other* than allergies and asthma? Do I need to order any tests to eliminate less common possibilities? Is the physical examination consistent with the history?" During the examination, I may think of additional questions I hadn't thought to ask before.

A complete description of a physical examination is beyond the scope of this book, but there are certain specific parts of the physical examination I always focus on:

Nose

It is not always possible to unequivocally differentiate between allergies and viral infections, but the presence and severity of inflammation in the nose is very important.

Throat

Many patients have signs of inflammation at the back of the throat, sometimes referred to as "cobblestoning." With practice it is possible to see back there in just a few seconds and get a feel for how much irritation there is, which usually results from either "above" (postnasal drip) or "below" (coming from the quite common condition of gastroesophageal reflux, referred to as GERD).

Extremities

Rashes and eczema frequently appear on arms and legs, and it is also important to inspect a child's nails and fingers. In addition to coloring of the nail beds, I always look for a relatively unusual shaping of the fingernails that has the unfortunate name of clubbing. This sign can be very subtle and is easily missed. If I am still uncertain, I sometimes ask to see a child's toenails, which catches everyone by surprise. This condition can be a sign of significant amounts of chronic, and sometimes silent, inflammation going on deep within the lungs, within the very smallest bronchial tubes. While clubbing can occur with asthma, it is unusual, and it does raise the possibility of more serious respiratory illnesses. Any child with clubbing merits more extensive testing.

If you check your child and think his nail beds may be "clubbed," don't panic. Clubbing can be perfectly normal and even run in families. It can also occur as a manifestation of chronic inflammation elsewhere in the body due to totally unrelated conditions. Only your doctor can assess whether the condition is a sign of anything else.

Chest

While listening with a stethoscope is helpful and important, it can also be misleading. One of the sentences I hate most is, "The chest is clear." A clear chest does not rule out significant asthma or bronchospasm. There may be no wheezing at all with as much as a 20 or even 30 percent reduction in the cross-sectional area of the airways, and wheezing may not occur with either severe asthma or severe pneumonia, when the airflow is so low that no sound is produced.

There is a lot more to a good chest exam than just using the stethoscope. Inspection for asymmetry, scoliosis (curvature of the spine), depth and rate of breathing, and the work of breathing, including the use of accessory muscles or so-called retractions, are all important parts of the physical exam. In fact, one of the single best pulmonary function tests, believe it or not, is how fast your child is breathing. Just about any lung disease will cause an increase in the respiratory rate, and there is an amazingly good correlation between the severity of the problem and the respiratory rate. Keep in mind that I am talking about a resting rate when a child is sitting quietly and not anxious or excited. This is not always possible in the frightening situation of an exam room, and the respiratory rate of a crying or frightened child can be very misleading.

STEP 3: DIAGNOSTIC TESTS

Many children will require no further testing after a complete history and physical examination. However, if there is any doubt as to the diagnosis, ancillary tests are important. Some primary care providers are comfortable with ordering and interpreting these tests, others would prefer to defer to either an allergy or pulmonary specialist.

Are You Satisfied?

If your child still doesn't seem to be doing well or you think something was missed, speak up. One or two visits to a specialist can often be enormously helpful. If further testing is required, some of the more common tests that may be done as part of an evaluation of your child are the following:

Allergy testing

There are a number of ways to test for allergies, and none are perfect. By far the best established methods are skin tests, and when done correctly, skin testing for allergies can be very helpful. Skin tests are usually done by allergists, and they must be done with care and attention to detail. If done improperly, the results can be very misleading. If your child is scheduled for skin tests, medications may affect the results. You will likely have been told to discontinue use of antihista-

mines for three to seven days before skin tests. This can be a
real problem for children in the midst of their allergy season.
A competent allergist will choose the tests to be done based
on the individual child's history and with knowledge of common triggers in that area.

COMMON ALLERGY TESTS

Specific Test	Other Names	Type	Advantages	Disadvantages
Scratch tests	Prick method	Skin	Simple to perform Relatively painless Many tests can be done at one visit Fairly sensitive and specific	May be frightening May miss true allergens, especially in young children
Intra-dermal Tests	Injection method	Skin	Most accurate and predictive of true allergic symptoms	Technique most important Time consuming
RAST tests	CAP RAST, in vitro	Blood	Easiest to perform Doesn't require an allergist	Least accurate and predictive of true allergic symptoms

Allergy skin tests, usually *scratch tests* or *prick tests*, are
fairly simple to perform, and they allow the doctor to test for
many allergens at one visit. The concept is to scratch the
skin with tiny amounts of possible allergens, and then watch
for an immediate IgE-mediated reaction, usually a small red
welt. This reaction usually occurs within about twenty min-

utes. In general, the larger the reaction, the more allergic your child is to that particular trigger. These tests are most often done on the back, where there is a large surface area of fairly uniform skin. Skin on the back may actually be preferable for allergy testing than skin on your child's arms or legs.

Children facing scratch or prick testing should be reassured the process won't be painful. Some kids start crying long before any testing has begun, and there is no consoling them. This makes the process much more unpleasant than necessary. Let your child know that most of the time he will only feel a very light scratching of the skin, nothing at all like shots he may have received.

There are other caveats with scratch tests: First, testing materials must be fresh and able to trigger a good reaction. Second, your child's skin must be able to react without overreacting. That's why it is important to place two control skin tests: One is a so-called *negative control*, which is to say, something that should not cause a reaction. The second is a *positive control*, usually histamine, which should definitely cause a reaction. If your child develops a reaction to the negative control or doesn't react to the positive control, then skin tests may not be interpretable.

Sometimes scratch testing is not workable when a child's overall skin reactions are generally slight. This is when an allergist may consider "intradermal" testing. (This is the same type of testing now used for tuberculosis.) In this method, the allergen is injected through a tiny needle into the top layer of the skin or dermis, creating a tiny bubble. Proper performance of these tests isn't easy. If the substance is placed too deep into the skin, the reaction will not be an accurate measure of the child's sensitivity. If an inadequate amount is planted, the child's reaction may be underestimated. This can be tricky, especially in young children who might not be totally convinced when they are told "this won't hurt." However, if done properly, intradermal testing is more sensitive than prick or scratch tests. In fact, since intradermal testing can detect very tiny allergic reactions, care must be taken not to overinterpret these tests.

The key to allergy testing is not who does the tests but how they are interpreted. Just because a child has a positive skin test to an allergen, that doesn't mean that particular trigger plays an important role in your child's symptoms. So, while allergy testing is useful, it can easily be misinterpreted or overinterpreted.

Blood tests

Parents and physicians are both attracted to newer blood tests for allergies, usually referred to as RAST (radioallergosorbent) tests. There are a number of variations on this theme, but they all are *in-vitro tests,* meaning instead of testing your child directly, you test a sample of their blood. Remember that if a person is allergic to something, they should have IgE molecules directed against that specific allergen floating in their bloodstream. Laboratories have figured out how to measure these tiny amounts of specific IgE, and this is simpler than performing skin tests. A sample of blood can be tested for dozens of allergens, with the results usually available in less than a week.

These tests are not as good as correctly performed skin tests. They are not as sensitive nor as specific, and they are more likely to miss true allergies or overestimate the importance of minor allergens. While not as good as skin tests, both primary care physicians and specialists find them helpful, particularly in young children on whom skin testing may be difficult. Ironically, these tests are the least accurate in young children.

One problem with allergy tests is the specificity of the tests. Just because a child reacts to a skin test or has specific IgE directed toward that allergen in a blood test, it doesn't mean a child will actually have symptoms when exposed to that specific allergen. This is particularly a problem with food allergy tests. While skin or RAST tests for food allergies can help guide your investigations, they rarely should be considered final.

Over the years, many alternative methods of allergy testing have been suggested and promoted. None of the alternatives listed below have been shown to be reliable:

- Sublingual provocation
- Electrodermal skin testing
- Cytotoxic food testing
- Hair analysis
- Food immune complex assays
- Iridology
- Video analysis of peripheral blood
- Serum IgG antibodies
- Elisa/ACT lymphocyte testing
- Neutralization testing

X-rays

If your child is not doing well, a chest X-ray can help rule out other causes of coughing or wheezing. Like any medical test, it is important not to order an X-ray unless for a specific reason. Don't be afraid to ask your physician why an X-ray is being requested, and how an X-ray may change your child's care.

When a child with asthma is completely well, they should have a completely normal X-ray, perfect in every way. Looking at an X-ray of a healthy child is like looking at the skin of a baby. Have you ever seen such perfection?

Unfortunately, our lungs are even more exposed to our environment than our skin. And just as we start to pick up all kinds of little scars and blemishes on our outside skin through life, our inside skin lining the bronchial tubes starts out smooth and unblemished, and, sad to say, it's all downhill after forty. About ten years ago, when I had to get a routine chest X-ray for a job, I took a look at my own films and thought they looked terrible. There were all kinds of "schmutz" throughout my lungs. I ran in panic to a radiologist and pushed my X-rays in front of him. He looked it over and said, "Normal."

"Normal?" I asked.

"Normal," he said. "Forty-year-old normal."

Unfortunately, I was only thirty-nine at the time!

The point of the story is your child's X-ray should be really crystal clear when they are perfectly well. And if it is perfect, you can be very reassured. During an exacerbation of asthma or bronchitis, the X-ray will often show mild evidence of bronchospasm, excess mucus production, and inflammation. For this reason I usually like to obtain a chest X-ray when children have been well for at least a few weeks.

X-rays are also sometimes ordered when a physician is considering the possibility of sinusitis. It's not always possible to diagnose sinusitis from physical examination alone. In fact, children hide sinusitis so well, that only for the last ten years have doctors understood how it is present in even very young children.

In teenagers and adults, regular old-fashioned sinus X-rays are sometimes adequate, but the best way to rule out sinus disease is with a CAT scan. Modern CAT scan machines use significantly less radiation than older models, but a sinus CAT scan still requires considerably more of it than plain films. So make sure your doctor has a good reason for ordering scans. When ordered appropriately, CAT scans of the sinuses can be enormously helpful. Ironically, sometimes they actually over-diagnose sinusitis.

Occasionally, CAT scans of the lungs are also ordered, and these really do give much more exquisite detail of the lungs and bronchial tubes than plain chest X-rays. I am concerned about everyone running around getting whole-body scans, looking for rare things. But I suppose over time the radiation exposure will continue to drop and the value will continue to increase. Who knows, maybe thirty years from now physicians will laugh at my insistence on a good old-fashioned chest X-ray.

Pulmonary Function Tests

Pulmonary function tests (PFTs) refer to a growing list of measurements made of your child's breathing. Some of these tests are very simple, such as the peak expiratory flow (PEF) that can be measured at home. Others, however, are quite complex and are only done at hospital-based pulmonary function laboratories.

Asthma causes a narrowing of the bronchial tubes, which is completely reversible. In between episodes, when a child with asthma is well, their lung function should be completely normal, as good as an Olympic athlete. In fact, that is one of the key goals for an asthma specialist to keep in mind. Unfortunately, there are many children with poorly controlled asthma whose lung function never gets back to perfect. This is bad. We now understand that in many children, chronic inflammation in the bronchial tubes can lead to a permanent "remodeling," or scarring, so that they are always narrowed. There are many immediate and long-term adverse effects of this chronic loss of lung function, a discussion of which could easily fill an entire chapter.

Key Point: ***Your children's lungs must last for their entire life. Do whatever you can to minimize any loss in lung function.***

The concept for a pulmonary function test is simple. While X-rays give you information about the *structure* of the lungs, PFTs give you information about the *function* of the lungs. This kind of information is important, and these tests are becoming increasingly common. Not too many years ago, these kinds of measurements were really only available at large medical centers. Now just about all asthma specialists, both allergists and pulmonologists, as well as an increasing number of primary care providers are using PFTs to help them manage all of their patients with asthma.

Most of these tests can only be performed by children old enough to cooperate, generally around four to six years of age. In the last few years, PFTs designed for infants and younger children have become available, but they are usually only done at children's hospitals or large pediatric pulmonology centers.

Here are quick descriptions of common pulmonary function tests:

PULMONARY FUNCTION TESTS

Specific Test	Advantages	Disadvantages
Peak Expiratory Flow (PEF)	Easy, inexpensive, good for the home	Not as accurate or reliable as more complicated tests; very effort-dependent

Spirometry	Perfect for office use, not as effort-dependent, gives more information than just a PEF	Too expensive for home use; still not great for children younger than three or four; not good for children with weak muscles
Complete PFTs	Most complete and accurate picture of all facets of lung function; many of the tests do not require much effort	Very expensive, time consuming; usually only available in hospitals; requires a very compulsive technician who carefully calibrates all equipment
Infant PFTs	Only way to measure lung function in children younger than three or children with weak respiratory muscles	Very new, not well standardized; only available at children's hospitals with dedicated pediatric pulmonary function labs

Peak Expiratory Flow (PEF)

Peak flow is the simplest and least expensive measurement. In fact, most asthma specialists will urge their patients with moderate or severe asthma to take home a peak-flow meter and use it to help manage their asthma. The peak expiratory flow (PEF) is exactly what it sounds like, the fastest flow rate you can generate while blowing into a tube. The bigger your lungs and bronchial tubes, the higher your PEF should be. Your physician will calculate the expected PEF for your child based on their age, height, and gender, and then you can compare your child's PEF to that predicted value. Just as there is a wide variability in normal weight or height, there is a wide variability in normal PEF. Your child's actual PEF is not as important as how it changes when they are ill.

Peak expiratory flow readings are helpful in determining when to start medications, when to back down off them, and very importantly, to make sure your child is truly getting back to perfect in between episodes. The first step is to establish your child's own "personal best" PEF when he is perfectly well. PEF will begin to drop as asthma worsens and return to baseline when asthma resolves. You may see a drop in PEF before any other signs of an impending exacerbation of asthma. So it is wise to insist your child measures their PEF on a regular basis. Then you can either start or increase medications quickly and prevent a significant attack.

Peak flow is a great tool, but it has limitations. There are other PFTs that are more sensitive or able to detect changes in your child's airways before PEF. Peak flow is also very effort-dependent, meaning it is not reliable in very young children who can't perform the required technique very well. It is also not as specific as other PFTs, meaning there are conditions other than asthma, such as postnasal drip and laryngitis, that may cause a drop in PEF. It is very important not to be fooled by the PEF, and never let it replace your own instincts as to how your child is doing.

Spirometry

Spirometry is a considerably more sensitive and specific measure of asthma severity. The results are much less dependent on your child's efforts and maturity, and I look forward to the day that inexpensive home spirometers are produced. The equipment is still quite expensive and complicated to use. Essentially all allergists and pulmonologists now have this equipment in their office and use these tests to monitor their patients. I am pleased to report that more and more primary care providers are purchasing this equipment and learning how valuable these numbers can be. Again, the major benefit of spirometry comes from checking your child's lung function when they are completely well, to be sure that they really get back to baseline after an attack.

Spirometry is less effort-dependent than PEF, but it is still limited to children older than three to six years of age, depending on their attention span and maturity.

Complete PFTs

If your child's diagnosis is unclear or his symptoms are difficult to control, the doctor may refer your child for a much more complete set of pulmonary function tests, usually done at a large medical center. Reassure your child that there are no needles involved. He will be asked to breathe into a variety of computerized devices, each designed to accurately measure different aspects of lung function.

These are expensive tests, often taking a couple of hours to complete. They are by far the most accurate way to be sure your child's lungs function normally. A more detailed discussion is beyond the scope of this chapter, but I do want to make one important point.

Complete PFTs do not require as much effort and cooperation from your child. The results are more dependent on the expertise of the technician who performs the tests. It is important that the laboratory has a lot of experience with children, particularly if your child is less than twelve years of age. Be very wary of a lab that predominantly studies adults. Be firm that your young child be studied in a lab dedicated to children.

Now and then we find other chronic conditions than can

mimic allergies and asthma. However, since 95 percent of the time there is no other problem, it is often difficult to decide when more extensive testing is appropriate. But if you feel your child's symptoms are not fully explained or adequately controlled, ask your physician if your child should have more extensive tests. The last thing you want is to find out after many years that serious illness has been missed. Again, some primary care physicians are comfortable making these decisions and ordering other tests, and some would prefer that a specialist get involved. There really are too many rare possibilities to go into in this chapter, but I thought I should mention a couple of the more commonly performed of these relatively less common tests.

Sweat test

There are only about 30,000 people in the United States with cystic fibrosis, a very serious illness, and the only absolute way to rule it out is with a *sweat test*. For this test, a freshly collected sample of your child's sweat is obtained by a number of slightly different methods. The test carries few risks, but it does take about an hour to complete. This test is difficult to perform. I urge you to only have a sweat test done at one of the approximately 115 cystic fibrosis care centers in the United States, accredited by the Cystic Fibrosis Foundation. That is the only way to be certain the results are reliable. The currently available blood tests for CF are not quite as good as a sweat test.

I remember one mother almost fainted when I mentioned a sweat test. It turns out her child, Walter, seems to have inherited his father's tendency to sweat like crazy. So she assumed Walter must have cystic fibrosis. Kids with CF do not sweat any more or less than anyone else. It's just that measurements need to be made of substances in the sweat. Don't panic if your child sweats a lot.

Immunological evaluation

Sometimes a child has classic signs and symptoms of allergies or asthma, and yet allergy testing is essentially negative. While your child still could have allergies, there are other abnormalities of the immune system that can mimic these conditions. A complete evaluation of the entire immune system is usually unnecessary, but deficiencies in one arm of your defenses, your child's antibodies, can mimic allergies or asthma or even be present in addition to allergies and asthma. For instance, a deficiency of an antibody called IgA is the most common immune deficiency of all, and this tends to leave children prone to chronic runny noses and ear and sinus infections, as well as coughing and wheezing. I frequently meet children who have been unsuccessfully treated for allergies for years before it was determined that allergies were not the true problem.

TAKE-HOME MESSAGES

- Many children can be adequately evaluated by their primary care provider based on a complete history and physical examination, with no other tests.

- Allergy tests are helpful in pinning down the actual triggers for your child's symptoms. Only by understanding the true triggers can you hope to prevent symptoms or plan appropriately.

- If your child is not doing well, or if doubt remains as to what exactly is going on, a specialist—allergist or pulmonologist—should be enlisted.

- X-rays and pulmonary function tests are important adjuncts to the complete evaluation of a child with suspected allergies or asthma.

- If allergies or asthma do not adequately explain your child's symptoms, then other less common causes for chronic illnesses must be considered and your physicians may recommend other tests, such as sweat tests or immunological evaluations.

SIX

Identifying Food Allergies

Food allergies are not as common as the popular press would have us believe, but for families coping with them, there are few things more frightening. Parents are understandably panicked about the potential threat to their child, and it's important to get advice on both the diagnosis and management of food allergies from an expert.

You may be somewhat heartened to learn that many people who think their child is allergic will actually find that this isn't the case. Food intolerances, such as abdominal cramping with ingestion of milk products, are common, but true food allergy is rare.

The most common symptoms of true food allergy are swelling of the lips, vomiting, diarrhea, hives, eczema, wheezing, or breathing problems. Though less common, food allergies can be life-threatening. One of the most frightening aspects, although rare, of food allergy is that a severe allergic reaction may occur even without actual ingestion of the specific food. There is the occasional anecdote of children developing reactions simply from being in a room in which the offending foods are being cooked.

The frequency of specific food allergies depends in part on the diet in that country. For instance, rice allergy is more common in Japan.

Key Point: *The most common food allergies are*
milk, eggs, fish, shellfish, tree nuts,
peanuts, wheat, and soy.

While the list of common food triggers is short, the actual edibles that cause problems are almost limitless, because almost all these foods can be found as ingredients in other dishes. This is just one of the reasons why diagnosis becomes so difficult.

Because of the complexity of the food we eat, families need to consult a specialist if a food allergy is suspected. With proper diagnosis, the family of the child who is merely intolerant can relax, knowing that the intolerance won't lead to a life-threatening reaction, and the child who is in danger if he has lunch at a table with someone eating peanut butter can be properly protected based on a definitive diagnosis.

Getting Help

Find an allergist or other healthcare provider experienced in the diagnosis and management of food allergies. Allergy tests can be very tricky to interpret. Knowing what to do with the information can be even tougher.

Diagnosis of Food Allergies in Infants

When food allergies are suspected in an infant, diagnosis is much easier because their intake is already so limited. If your baby is on a formula from cow's milk, the doctor may suggest a switch to either breast milk exclusively or to another formula. The most common alternatives are formulas based on soy protein. Changing your baby's formula will tell you and your doctor a great deal about what is going on with your child.

The problem is that some kids who are allergic to cow's milk also develop allergic symptoms to soy protein, and vice versa, so if that doesn't work, your doctor may try one of the "elemental" formulas, which almost never trigger allergic reactions. These formulas are expensive, harder to find, and some infants don't seem to like their taste, so it's great if the problem can be resolved with one simple switch.

You need to give this process time. Symptoms may continue for days or even weeks after removal of the offending allergen. Not too long ago I met a lovely couple, Paula and Phil, with their very cranky and gassy four-month-old, Patty. (I think Patty's older siblings are Peter and Priscilla.) They started with Enfamil, switched to Isomil, then worked their way through Similac, Prosobee, and the more elemental formulas Nutramigen and Pregestimil, all within three weeks—without success. This was clearly not the way to go. If you change formulas, stick with it for a few weeks. If your baby is still symptomatic, consider a more thorough medical evaluation, possibly by a pediatric gastroenterologist. Keep in mind that allergy is by no means the only reason for formula intolerance.

Although your baby cannot be allergic to breast milk, there have been cases of babies having reactions to the tiny amount of proteins in breast milk from the mother's diet. This sometimes explains why very rarely a baby seems to have an allergic reaction the first time they eat something like peanut butter. All of the common food allergens—that is, the proteins from eggs, peanuts, tree nuts, wheat, cow's milk, and soy—can pass into breast milk, usually about two to six hours after a mother ingests the food in question. If you suspect your infant is reacting to substances in breast milk, it is well worth discussing with a physician.

Diagnosis of Food Allergies in Children

The first step your physician will take is to obtain a careful history. Keeping a food diary is helpful (see page 105). Be prepared to answer these questions:

What were the specific symptoms that caused concern?
In older kids and adults, hives and wheezing are the most common symptoms. But infants and young children sometimes manifest food allergies as colic, poor growth, crankiness, and even occasionally blood in their stools.

What was the timing of the reaction?
Most food allergies occur within an hour after eating the food in question, though there are exceptions.

Did your child consume a lot of one particular food?
Sometimes the severity of the reaction is related to the amount of food eaten.

Did an allergy medicine help the reaction?
For example, antihistamines should have relieved hives that were caused by a food allergy.

Did anyone else develop reactions at the same time?
If other people had reactions, then the reaction was not likely a true food allergy.

If the suspected food is fish, was it well cooked?
Or was it raw or undercooked? Allergens are often destroyed in fish with complete cooking. So sometimes kids can eat well-cooked fish without a problem, but have allergic reactions when the fish is rare.

One tricky situation concerning fish is that some fish are actually contaminated with histamine, the chemical that triggers allergic reactions. In that case the symptoms will certainly appear allergic in nature though the child isn't allergic to the fish itself.

Were other foods ingested at the same time?
This may confuse the picture because the allergic reactions might be to something other than the food you suspect. Also, if there is lots of food in the stomach, sometimes this delays *gastric emptying*, meaning the absorption of allergens into the bloodstream, and therefore any allergic symptoms may be delayed.

Keeping a Food Diary

If your child has had a violent reaction to a food, then see a doctor right away. If the symptoms are vague (crankiness) or, for example, hives or eczema, then keeping a food diary for a couple of weeks can be very helpful. Buy a notebook for this purpose so that everything can be recorded by date and in an orderly manner. Write down everything your child eats or drinks, and any associated symptoms.

Whenever possible, note brand names and all of the ingredients in processed foods. Sometimes the culprit is not the food itself but other additives or ingredients, such as sulfite preservative, monosodium glutamate (a flavor enhancer), and tartrazine, also known as FD&C Yellow No. 5 (a food color). The Food and Drug Administration recently discovered that in spite of strict labeling laws, as many as 25 percent of manufacturers fail to list common ingredients that may cause potentially fatal allergic reactions, *so you need to be cautious when trying new packaged foods.*

Testing for Food Allergies

Like testing for any other type of allergy, testing for a food allergy begins with a complete history and physical examination, followed by skin or blood (RAST) tests, and usually then requires food elimination or a medically supervised food challenge.

If a suspected food allergen is eliminated from the diet and there is an unequivocal improvement in symptoms, there is still no definitive diagnosis. It is almost impossible to eliminate just one food item at a time, and the improvement could be a coincidence. If the food is then reintroduced and symptoms increase, it is suspicious but still can be very misleading. Unfortunately, there are still many confounding variables that can fool parents and physicians alike.

CONSIDER AN ELIMINATION DIET

Elimination diets are best overseen by a doctor to be sure the diet is properly designed. Eliminating a food sounds simple enough, but your child still needs a balanced diet. And symptoms are sometimes delayed or linger longer than you might expect. Or symptoms may resolve on their own, so the diagnosis is only confirmed when you carefully add the food back and symptoms return. This process can get very confusing, so I don't recommend you do this on your own. The most important reason for relying on a professional to orchestrate an elimination diet has to do with the "adding back" step. If you add back a food to which your child is allergic, the reaction can be dangerous.

DOUBLE-BLIND FOOD CHALLENGES

The gold standard of testing for a food allergy is what is known as a *double-blind food challenge*. The suspected food is disguised so neither the patient, their family, nor the testers actually know for sure whether your child has ingested the actual food or a look-alike placebo. This kind of testing can be very helpful, but it is time-consuming, expensive, and may have significant risk in children who are highly allergic.

In this type of testing, the foods in question must be hidden in something else so that neither tester nor child knows which food is under scrutiny. (Hence the term double-blind.) This way the test is totally objective. In older children who can swallow capsules, the doctor will hide small amounts of each food in opaque capsules and ask your child to swallow them one at a time. Hiding the foods is trickier for young children who don't like to swallow pills, but the foods can sometimes be buried into mushy foods.

As you can imagine, this is the best way to correctly identify specific food allergens. However, this should almost never be done with a food to which your child already had a severe reaction. And it is obviously very important that anyone performing these tests be well prepared to handle any allergic reactions that may occur.

EXERCISE-INDUCED FOOD ALLERGY

This relatively unusual type of allergic reaction can be very difficult to diagnose. Kids who suffer from this problem can often eat a certain food most of the time without any reaction. But if they exercise after eating a specific food, they begin to itch or develop hives, they may get light-headed, and they can even have a full-blown anaphylactic reaction. The increased metabolic rate and increased body temperature associated with exercise accentuates the allergic reaction. If your child puts off exercise for a couple of hours after eating the specific food, the problem is solved.

Controversial Aspects of Food Allergies

One of the longest living theories is that hyperactivity in children is due to food allergies. Occasionally there are children who are sensitive to preservatives and other additives in processed foods, especially if ingested in large quantities. And I'm sure that a child who is itchy, wheezing, sneezing, or drowsy from allergy medications won't have the greatest attention span in school. Certainly huge quantities of caffeine from soda, coffee, or tea can make anyone twitchy. However, by and large, true food allergies do not explain this tremendous problem.

Other symptoms are sometimes thought to be due to food allergies, but probably aren't. The number one example is migraine headaches. Histamine and other chemicals in food can certainly trigger headaches, but very few true migraines are due to food allergies. I have heard of the expression "cerebral allergy," occasionally used to explain the reason for feeling anxious or depressed or having trouble concentrating. I can find no data to support this theory. But older people are convinced that their arthritis is made worse by certain foods and there really is no evidence for this either.

No Definitive Diagnosis?

If a diagnostic evaluation fails to pin down specific food triggers, keep looking for connections. While it is rare, even fruits and vegetables can cause food allergies, but the more likely culprit is one of the more commonly known allergenic foods, possibly disguised in some processed food. If your child appears to be having intermittent symptoms such as hives, without an easy explanation, try to think about what they may have eaten, drunk, or been exposed to in the preceding hour or so.

Many years ago, sixteen members of my family drove together for a two-week trip through parts of the southwest United States. Two of my nephews, ages eight and ten, often grew bored and spent a few minutes at every stop kicking around a hackysack. They were getting pretty good, but I can't say the adults in the group were all that upset when my brother's son, Mark, kicked it into a tree. That was that. Mark frequently has allergies and eczema and occasionally breaks out in hives, but low and behold, Mark's mother noticed that he stopped having hives in the middle of the trip. She didn't think to associate the event with the lost hackysack. Then, a couple of days later, Mark convinced his dad to buy him another hackysack, and all of a sudden the hives started reappearing. It turns out the crunchy feel and sound associated with that hackysack was due to crushed nut shells inside.

In a later chapter on prevention of food allergies, I will review some of the other less obvious substances that may contain allergens. For instance, cheeses or mortadella may contain nuts. In fact, tree nuts such as walnuts, almonds, and pecans find themselves in all sorts of places.

TAKE-HOME MESSAGES

- If you suspect food allergies, it is really important to accurately pin them down.

- Food allergies almost never cause *chronic* asthma symptoms.

- Food diaries can be very helpful.

- Skin or blood tests for food allergies can be misleading and need careful interpretation by a physician with experience and expertise in this area.

- Elimination diets should be done only with the supervision of a physician.

- Severe reactions to foods are fortunately rare.

PART THREE:

ALLERGY AND ASTHMA ACTION PLAN: PREVENTION

SEVEN

Allergy Shots:
Who, What, When,
Where, Why, and How

"Why don't you just give her allergy shots?"
is a question you might get from friends
when your child is sniffing and sneezing. It's a logical question without an easy answer. Or you may hear the opposite opinion: "Oh, allergy shots don't work, everyone knows that." So what's the deal with allergy shots? Do they work or don't they, and when should you consider them?

Allergy shots have been available for a long time, yet we still don't completely understand why they work. *Immunotherapy,* the medical term for allergy shots, is based on the observation that people may sometimes develop a tolerance to an allergen if they are gradually exposed to increasing amounts. A child is injected with gradually increasing amounts of the actual proteins to which he is allergic—an amount so small that no significant reaction occurs. The goal is to desensitize the immune system so that your child can now withstand exposure to higher doses of that specific allergen without significant symptoms.

Immunotherapy has the potential to minimize your

child's symptoms without constant medication. This approach, while helpful, is expensive, time-consuming, and not without risk—and there is no guarantee of benefit. Most allergists would agree that if your child's symptoms can be controlled safely with well-tolerated medications such as antihistamines and nasal sprays, allergy shots are probably not worth the bother.

Key Point: ***Insist on a board-certified allergist,***
an expert in immunotherapy.

When Immunotherapy Is Most Helpful

Allergy shots can only prevent reactions against specific proteins. They work best when a specific allergen can be identified. Allergy shots will not be effective if your child's symptoms are due to viral infections or nonspecific irritants, such as dust or pollution.

WHICH CONDITIONS CAN BE TREATED WITH ALLERGEN IMMUNOTHERAPY?

Allergic rhinitis	Yes
Allergic conjunctivitis	Yes
Asthma	Yes, in selected patients
Food allergies	No
Insect allergies	Yes
Atopic dermatitis	No
Urticaria (hives)	No
Pet allergies	Maybe

ALLERGIC RHINITIS

The most common reason for allergy shots is allergic rhinitis (hay fever). If your child's symptoms are predominantly triggered by inhaled environmental allergens such as trees, grasses, weeds, dust mites, and molds, then allergy shots may be the right solution.

ALLERGIC CONJUNCTIVITIS

Every spring my office fills with kids suffering with red and itchy eyes, a particular problem if you are allergic to trees and grass. An almost irresistible urge to rub your eyes can often lead to secondary infection. What a mess. Contact lens are usually out of the question when eye allergies flair. There are a variety of medications that can really help, but take it from someone who knows personally, allergic conjunctivitis can be very difficult to control. Allergy shots may help, though most families won't choose years of shots for eye allergies alone.

ASTHMA

Allergists and pulmonologists have long debated the benefits of allergy shots for asthma. Studies done in the past failed to show significant benefit. Immunotherapy will only work if your child's symptoms are in large part caused by a limited number of known allergens. If your child's asthma is triggered by viral infections or exercise, allergy shots will be ineffective. In highly allergic children, immunotherapy may only protect against some of the sensitivities.

Many pulmonologists remain cynical about this approach for asthma. However, the immunotherapy process has greatly improved, and allergists have become much more experienced at identifying asthmatic patients for whom immunotherapy will be helpful.

Some children develop significant wheezing or shortness of breath in response to immunotherapy, making it difficult if not impossible to increase the tolerated dose of allergens. If you notice your child develops coughing or wheezing one to two days after every shot, call your allergist. The plan will need to be slowed down or discontinued.

Given these considerations, most allergists recommend allergy shots in children with asthma only if they also have significant allergic rhinitis and their asthma is under good control.

FOOD ALLERGIES

Allergy shots have not been proven to work for children with food allergies. Severe food allergies are so frightening that many alternative forms of immunotherapy have been touted as effective. You may hear about aromatherapy, homeopathy, acupuncture, naturopathy, herbal medicine, chelation therapy (a blood "cleansing" therapy), and Ayurvedic medicine (an ancient Indian form of holistic medicine that is actually a nice addition to conventional therapy). These are just a few of the ways people have tried to deal with food allergies. I have never run across any substantiating data supporting these approaches.

It would be wonderful if children could be desensitized against foods that have triggered severe or anaphylactic reactions. There are some exciting research efforts directed at developing allergy shots for foods, but they still seem to be years away. Until these methods are proven safe and effective in large, carefully designed clinical trials, the only current approach to food allergies is to avoid eating the offending foods.

INSECT ALLERGIES

Protecting children who have had severe allergic reactions to insect stings is one of the best uses of allergy shots. Experts universally agree that venom immunotherapy is important and potentially lifesaving. Effectiveness has been proven for honeybees, hornets, wasps, and yellow jackets. In recent years, imported fire ants have been added to the list of causes for severe allergic reactions, and immunotherapy against fire ants can be effective. Allergy shots are effective against certain biting insects, such as the blood-sucking arthropod *Triatoma protracta,* and perhaps against inhaled insect allergens from cockroaches and certain types of houseflies.

SKIN ALLERGIES

Atopic dermatitis (eczema) and chronic hives (urticaria) can be very disabling conditions for children. Unfortunately, immunotherapy is of little use in these situations.

PETS

Will allergy shots permit your family to get a pet? Excellent allergists disagree on the value of immunotherapy against dog or cat dander. Some kids seem to benefit and others not so much. Minimizing exposure to the offending allergens is preferable.

Making the Decision

I usually don't recommend allergy shots before age five, though there are exceptions, such as a child who has had a severe allergic reaction to insect stings. Then steps to protect against an allergic reaction may need to be taken as soon as possible.

There is no point in starting immunotherapy unless both parent and child are willing to make the time commitment to follow through and keep up with the schedule. One day a patient of mine with asthma, sixteen-year-old MaryAnn, was in my office complaining about her allergies. I had referred her to an allergy specialist five years before who had begun allergy shots without much benefit. As we talked, the reason became clear: She had missed more than half of her appointments with the allergist. "Why?" I asked. It turns out she was just too busy. She is on the swim team, takes ballet, and is in cheerleading. She helps out at her church on weekends and is now taking driving lessons. She is in five other clubs at school and goes away to summer camp for eight weeks. Allergy shots are not for everyone.

On the other hand, I should also tell you about Beth and Amanda. These girls are twelve-year-old twins who have been my patients for many years. They look identical to me, but I am well aware that they aren't exactly alike: Amanda suffers from terrible allergies. Despite all kinds of prescriptions, she suffers every spring from terrible headaches and sinus infections, sometimes sneezing for an hour each morning. High doses of antihistamines dry her out too much, and decongestants make her heart race. For Amanda, allergy shots made sense. Beth is more fortunate. Various combinations of medicines control her symptoms, at least most of the year. In May, when trees and grasses are both pollinating, her allergies sometimes act up, but so far allergy shots haven't seemed worth it.

Key Point: ***Allergy shots should be considered
if medications are inadequate.***

Selecting the Right Allergens

Immunotherapy must be tailored to each individual. Your child's allergist should ask about your environment, assessing all possible indoor and outdoor allergens that may be affecting your child. (Refer to Chapter 5 for complete information on the diagnostic process.) He should be knowledgeable about local and regional allergens in your geographical area, including any new allergens such as plants and trees recently introduced into the area. Accurate allergy tests must then be performed to help guide the process.

The most commonly used allergens for allergy shots are dust mites, animal allergens, mold spores, and the pollens of weeds, trees, and grasses. If the doctor chooses too many allergens, you may not get the desired protective benefit from individual allergens. And of course, if allergens left out are significant triggers for your child's symptoms, you may be disappointed in the results. These are key decisions that can make all of the difference.

Whenever possible, allergists should try to use standardized allergenic extracts that have defined and consistent potencies. This should decrease the likelihood of triggering significant allergic reactions as the dose is increased. Sometimes non-standardized extracts must be used, and these are trickier since the potency may vary between lots of the same product. If your child starts shots at one facility and must be switched to another office, this is important to remember. Suddenly the same apparent dose of allergen may cause a significantly greater reaction.

Your child's allergist needs to be compulsive about how the extracts are handled or the potency will fade and you may waste time. Potency is not only determined by the concentration of actual allergen in the vial, but the passage of time and the temperature at which they are stored. Aqueous extracts should be refrigerated at 4° Celsius, and only sit out at room temperature for brief periods of time. Some of the extracts arrive in a lyophilized dry powder to maintain potency on the shelf. It is important that these dry allergens be reconstituted carefully, adding the correct amount of stabilizing agents to the diluted vials. Attention to detail is very important. In the past, some allergy extracts were mixed in vegetable or mineral oil to try and slow the release of allergen at the site of injection and decrease the risk of immediate allergic reactions. These can cause serious side effects and should no longer be used. Some allergists use extracts that are absorbed to alum, a process that slows the release of the allergen into the skin, again with the goal of slowing any local allergic reaction. This is approved and available; though allergists do not all agree whether this really matters. If your child is having significant local redness or swelling with allergy shots, ask your allergist if different kinds of extracts should be considered.

It remains controversial whether it is just as effective to mix various allergy extracts together in the same vial or if they need to remain separate. Some products have significant amounts of proteolytic enzymes that may cause other allergens in the mix to lose their potency. Ask your child's allergist how he or she feels about these issues, and what your child is actually receiving. Most people seem to be unaware of these details. With this knowledge, you will be able to discuss these issues with your child's doctor if the shots don't seem to be helping or there are unacceptable allergic reactions from the shots.

Allergy Shots: The Routine

Most children are initially treated with one or two injections per week. The frequency of injections decreases once high maintenance doses are reached.

The proper duration of therapy is somewhat controversial

and really has to be tailored to each child. With the standard schedule, allergy shots need to be given for at least eight to twelve months to be beneficial. If a child does not improve significantly within that time, the plan should be reevaluated. Perhaps different allergens should be selected.

If a child's condition improves by the end of the first year, two at the latest, most allergists would recommend that maintenance doses be continued for another three or four years. Usually your child will remain well protected for many years. Sometimes, however, the protective effect wears off soon after discontinuing the shots.

Your allergist may recommend repeat allergy tests along the way, since as your child is desensitized, repeat allergy testing may turn negative or the size of the skin reaction may decrease. However, many allergists find little benefit from frequent repeat testing, since allergy tests are not perfect predictors of actual symptoms anyway.

For bee sting and other insect venom immunotherapy, most allergists recommend continuing treatment for at least five years, and then trying to stop and see what happens. Optimally, you want to see that your child no longer has a positive skin test or blood test (specific IgE) to the venom you have been using. This may not always occur.

Are They Safe?

Allergy shots are quite safe. However, since the allergist is injecting the actual protein that is known to trigger allergic reactions into your child, it is not too surprising that children can develop allergic symptoms as the dose is gradually increased. This is where you need to be certain that you are going to an allergist with lots of pediatric experience. Safe escalation of the dose in allergy shots is rather an art. Nonetheless, the incidence of significant reactions is rare.

Death from an anaphylactic reaction is extraordinarily un-likely, but it has been reported. That is another reason why you should insist that all appropriate precautions are taken (see below).

SAFETY PRECAUTIONS FOR GIVING ALLERGY SHOTS

- Allergy shots should not be given at all to patients considered at higher risk for reactions. Most of these contraindications apply predomi-nantly to adults: patients taking medicines known as beta-blockers; patients with significant high blood pressure or heart, liver, or kidney disease; anyone who is pregnant. Even these kinds of high-risk patients may be treated if there is a dangerous unavoidable exposure that necessitates taking this risk.

- The person prescribing the allergy shots should be either an allergist-immunologist or someone expertly trained in this form of therapy.

- Make sure the office is properly equipped to handle any allergic reactions, including the fortunately rare occurrence of anaphylaxis.

- The shots should be given under supervision of your allergist or someone trained to recognize the early signs and symptoms of anaphylaxis and know what to do in an emergency. In the past, the allergist commonly made up the allergy materials, but your primary care provider gave the shots. The potency of allergy shots has improved, and so has the risk of an allergic reaction. While some primary care providers are experienced and equipped to safely administer allergy shots, most children in the United States receive their shots at their allergist's office.

- Children who are acutely ill with an infection or asthma should not receive an allergy shot, which could make them worse.

- Since so many children with allergies have asthma, it is very important that their asthma be under good control. This is sometimes a catch-22: If allergies are the reason for poorly controlled asthma, a patient may not be safely desensitized until his asthma is better. Your child may actually require more asthma medicines while they are undergoing allergy immunotherapy. Better safe than sorry. Measuring pulmonary function can be invaluable. Since most asthmatic children who are receiving allergy shots are old enough to perform tests such as spirometry, I recommend that the allergist routinely check lung function before each shot.

- Don't rush out of the office with your child. Most allergists will insist that your child wait a minimum of twenty minutes or longer after each injection.

Rush Desensitization

To achieve desensitization more rapidly, some doctors will give injections on a daily regimen, often referred to as rush desensitization. Occasionally, what is known as a rapid rush method is used. In very sick children who are hospitalized and in desperate need of a specific antibiotic to which they are allergic, a child may receive an increased dose every one or two hours. The faster you escalate the dose, the higher the risks of significant side effects. Because of this risk, the rapid rush method is usually performed in the hospital. There are very few reasons to attempt the rapid rush method.

Allergists have long sought safe and effective alternatives to allergy shots, including topical placement of allergens in the nose, inhaled into the lungs, given orally, or placed under the tongue. None of these are ready to be made available to consumers.

Anti-IgE Therapy

This is a completely new kind of therapy just becoming available, and as of this writing, it is hard to know how this approach will fit in. Two products have been studied and one of them, Xolair, is now out on the market. This medication is a high-tech marvel given by injection every two or four weeks. The formula consists of molecules that attach to any IgE circulating in the bloodstream, theoretically preventing allergic reactions against pretty much anything.

Since this medication is expensive and we don't have any long-term experience, anti-IgE therapy is now only being used for patients with moderate to severe asthma triggered by allergies that cannot be well controlled with the usual medications. In the near future we will start learning how effective this therapy is, and I suspect we will soon consider this approach for children who have had serious allergic reactions to foods, insects, or other potentially devastating triggers.

TAKE-HOME MESSAGES

- Not all children with allergies or asthma need allergy shots.

- Allergy shots can be helpful, particularly in children older than age five in whom medications have been inadequate.

- Allergy shots take significant time and commitment to be successful.

- Make sure an expert in immunotherapy, usually an allergist-immunologist, prescribes your child's allergy shots.

- Make sure the facility your child is going to is well equipped and staffed for unexpected emergencies.

- If your child has asthma as well as allergies, make sure their asthma is under good control before they receive an injection.

- If allergy shots don't seem to have made much of a difference within at most one or two years, rethink them.

EIGHT

Day-to-Day Prevention
at Home and Beyond

Avoiding allergic triggers is far better than either chronic medications or allergy shots; however, convincing parents to follow through with preventive strategies is not easy. The reality is that prevention is difficult, treatment seems easy. In this chapter I will describe ways to minimize dust and dust mites in your child's bedroom. These are of proven benefit, yet many parents have not been able to complete these steps.

Parents of children with severe allergies sometimes go to the opposite extreme, becoming so anxious about environmental exposures that their child's world becomes smaller and smaller, a cocoon of fear. Susanna, age ten, has significant allergies and asthma, but she hasn't had any major problems since she first came to me after a hospitalization at age five. Susanna herself is a very relaxed and confident child, but her mom still lives daily with intense anxiety that her daughter will suffer another severe attack. Right now the big issue concerns sleepovers. While her girlfriends are more than welcome to sleep over at her house, Susanna is not permitted to sleep elsewhere, and after turning down many offers, her girlfriends have stopped asking.

As in so many areas of parenting, I believe the key is to learn as much as you can, then find a *moderate* approach that makes sense to you and your family.

Key Point: ***Minimizing exposure to allergens is difficult work, but it is well worth the effort.***

Secondary Prevention of Allergies and Asthma

Once a child is sensitized to an allergen, is it possible to prevent that child from developing severe allergic symptoms or asthma? If so, this is an argument for early allergy testing of children. If a child has a positive skin or blood test for a specific allergen, it seems reasonable to focus attention on decreasing environmental exposure to that allergen, even if your child doesn't seem to currently show any symptoms. For instance, a child may test positive for dogs and cats even though her symptoms don't seem particularly worse when she is around a cat or dog. Perhaps decreasing her exposure might decrease the likelihood of her eventually developing significant allergy symptoms or asthma later on. Honestly, no one knows for sure whether these steps would significantly benefit your child.

So what do I advise? Use common sense. If your child tests positive for dog or cat allergies or just seems very prone to allergies in general, it really doesn't seem logical to bring a new furry pet into your home. And if you already have a dearly beloved dog or cat, minimize your child's exposure by keeping the animal out of your child's bedroom. Or if your pet is getting on in years, don't replace him right away. But unless your dog or cat is causing very significant symptoms, I don't think you necessarily have to find a new home for the heartthrob of the family. I learned a long time ago that most pet owners will get rid of their asthma or allergy doctor long before they get rid of their pet.

Even more aggressive approaches at secondary prevention are being tried but cannot yet be recommended. For instance, for many children, one of the first signs that they may be destined to be atopic, or prone to allergies or asthma, is eczema. Two studies have suggested that giving antihistamines to these children may decrease the likelihood they will start wheezing. Another study suggests that giving allergy shots to children with positive allergy tests but no current symptoms may prevent future asthma. These studies are intriguing, but we clearly need more data before suggesting these approaches.

Hands-On Solutions to Reducing Allergies and Asthma (Tertiary Prevention)

The remainder of this chapter will discuss the avoidance of known triggers, including indoor and outdoor allergens, drugs, and pollutants.

AVOIDANCE OF INDOOR ALLERGENS

The first place to start is in your child's bedroom, since that is the room where he spends the most time, but you can't stop there. Keep in mind kids spend a lot of time in the family room, the den, and the kitchen, too; so you really have to think about all of those areas.

There is another increasingly important living space many parents do not consider—the inside of your car. Like adults, many children spend a good portion of their day in the family car where the air quality can be really bad. As we review steps you can take around your home, consider which of these might apply to your automobile. For example, clean and vacuum your car regularly—and no smoking!

DUST MITES

The number one indoor allergen is the infamous dust mite. This tiny varmint, microscopically small, looks kind of like a minuscule spider. It likes to live in dark, warm, and humid environments, such as in your mattresses and pillows. These creatures are everywhere, and their debris are potent allergens. They love to eat our dander (flakes of dead skin), and while we can't really hope to get rid of them completely, we definitely can reduce a child's exposure.

Here are some steps to take that can make a big difference to your child:

MEASURES FOR REDUCING EXPOSURE TO DUST MITES

- Encase mattresses, box springs, pillows, and comforters in mite-proof covers.
- Wash all bedding in hot water (130° Fahrenheit).
- Avoid carpeting, upholstered furniture, and other dust-catching items.
- Avoid high humidity.
- Vacuum with double-thick bags, optimally with HEPA filters.
- Replace curtains with washable shades or curtains.
- Frequently clean or change filters in hot-air heating units.

- Avoid down or feather comforters. They look tempting in catalogs, but really can do a number on your nose and bronchial tubes. Stick to washable blankets or comforters.

- Encase pillows, mattresses, box springs, and comforters in mite-proof covers. The concept is simple: Place a barrier between your child's nose and the dust mites. These mattress covers are usually a blend of cotton and polyester and have a vinyl back. They are easily obtained at department stores, bedding supply stores, on-line, or by mail order and are well worth it. More mites will gradually build up on the outside surface of these covers, so they must be cleaned periodically— vacuum them monthly since taking them on and off frequently is a pain. If you really can't part with your comforter, at least encase it in a good allergy barrier. Then you can put the encased comforter in a duvet if you'd like.

- Wash all bedsheets and blankets in hot water. All bedsheets should be washed in very hot water. Dust mites die in water that is 130° Fahrenheit or higher. Unfortunately, this is sometimes easier said than done. (Many washing machines limit the water temperature.) Repeated hot water washing will certainly shorten the life of your sheets and pillowcases. Blankets should be washed frequently as well, so buy ones that can go in the machine.

- Avoid dust ruffles on your child's bed. Any additional decoration on a bed—from pillow shams to bedspreads, dust ruffles, and canopies—are a great hiding place for dust mites. Your child with allergies and asthma should sleep in a bed where everything is easily washable.

- Avoid thick carpeting. Consider removing wall-to-wall carpeting from bedrooms. If you can't have hardwood floors, select low-pile carpeting and limit clutter so you can easily and effectively vacuum the carpeting on a regular basis.

- Take a look at window treatments. Try to avoid fancy decorative drapes. Washable shades or curtains are the best choice. Venetian blinds are really tough to vacuum effectively and most people really don't have the time or energy to keep up with the dust.

- Remember that stuffed animals are just lovable dust catchers. If your child must sleep with a teddy bear or a well-hugged stuffed dog, okay, but keep the numbers from growing—one or two stuffed animals seem to multiply, and the next thing you know your child has a full menagerie. Like most parents, I suppose, we didn't really pay much attention as the stuffed zoo expanded over the years. Eventually, we found there was barely any room for our daughter amongst the dolls, bears, and rabbits. Limit your child to one or two special friends in bed, and if he or she has a collection elsewhere in the room, vacuum it.

- Set a limit on clutter, including dropped clothing. Clothing also collects dust, so encourage your child not to leave clothing strewn throughout the room. Of course, now that my daughter is almost eighteen we've lost complete control over her room, and I can't even remember the last time I saw the floor peeking out from between her clothes. (Maybe you'll do better.) Certainly, with young children firmer limits are possible— few young children must try on several outfits before leaving in the morning.

- Dust frequently, but not when your child is in the room. Start from the top and work down. Then take a break and let the dust settle for about fifteen or twenty minutes before vacuuming up the dust that has dropped to the bed and floor.

- Vacuum regularly. Vacuuming is important but must be done wisely. Vacuum cleaners are supposed to retain dust and dust mites in the bag, but many actually spew them back into the air. The vacuums that are best at controlling dust are those that use a double bag system or that have a good small particle filter system, such as a HEPA (high efficiency particulate air) filter, built in. If you're not yet in the market for a new vacuum, there are steps you can take that can improve the process using your current machine: Make sure the bag within your vacuum cleaner is reasonably empty when you vacuum the bedrooms. As the bag fills up, more dust will be sprayed into the room, so start in the bedroom if possible. Try to get good bags that trap dust mites. If you have difficulty finding these products, ask your allergist or pulmonologist. There are excellent mail-order and Internet allergy supply companies.

- Take a good look at your heating system. Forced-hot-air heating is very popular, but it also serves to blow a great deal of dust around. Most of these systems have either washable or disposable filters in the system, which should be changed or cleaned before the heat is turned on and every month throughout the heating season. If the filter is disgusting when you change it, change it more often in the future. Central electrostatic filtering systems can be added to most heating or air-conditioning systems, eliminating the need for changing filters, but they can be expensive. Good central filtering is important, but the air blows through the ductwork and finally out into the room. Service companies will vacuum out ducts, and if you've had construction done recently or live in an older home, it's worth the investment. In addition, consider placement of filters over air vents that go directly into the bedrooms. These can usually be obtained at a good hardware store. If you have radiators instead, you are in luck.

- Don't allow the humidity in your home to be too high. Dust mites like humidity. In the winter, many people hate the feeling of dry heat, but try not to let the relative humidity remain above 40 to 45 percent. It is usually not necessary to measure humidity in your home unless your home has a particular problem with moisture. In that case you can buy an inexpensive hygrometer, but I am concerned it may not always be accurate.

Key Point: *Humidifiers are rarely a good idea.*
They're a great place for mold and
bacteria to grow and dust mites
thrive in humid environments.

- Consider HEPA filters for your home, but only as a last resort. Unless you live in a particularly dusty home, adding room-sized HEPA filters shouldn't be necessary if you've taken the other recommended steps. However, if your child is still suffering from dust mite–related symptoms despite all of your efforts, then a good HEPA filter may help. If you do purchase one, make sure it is powerful enough to clean the intended room.

- What about negative ion generators? Some home devices include ionizers that add a slightly negative charge to the air. This approach decreases the amount of soot and other particulate matter in the air, particularly from tobacco smoke. Tobacco smoke smells also apparently decrease. However, there is almost no unbiased information about any of the health benefits of these devices. For instance, there are many other chemicals in cigarette smoke not removed by ion generators, and these chemicals may be far worse than the pollutants you can see or smell.

- Historically, one way to breathe ionized and purified air was to travel to subterranean salt mines or caves, in which the air is rich in microscopic salt particles. Home air purifiers that use salt may hold great promise.

- What about ozone generators? Some air-filtration systems produce ozone. These devices have many proponents, but the Environmental Protection Agency cautions there is very little unbiased data supporting their use, and you cannot assume that home devices, even when used according to manufacturer's recommendations, will keep ozone levels at low and safe concentrations. Don't forget the rule of unintended consequences: My general instinct is that adding chemicals to our environment is rarely the best way to go.

MOLD SPORES

There are some specific steps that will reduce mold in and around your home.

MEASURES FOR REDUCING EXPOSURE TO MOLD SPORES

- Limit water leaks in your house.

- Control mildew in wet areas such as kitchens or bathrooms by using bleach or other antifungal products, particularly in showers and on windowsills.

- Keep the humidity less than 45 percent.

- Reduce mold on the outside of your home.

- Avoid plants in bedrooms.

  - Basements are often the source of the problem. If water gets into your basement, mold grows, so try to keep it dry. This may mean repairing small leaks or being certain that the house foundation is strong. While mold can be killed with bleach or other anti-fungal agents, very few people can keep up with it. A mold problem in the basement is particularly acute if you have forced-hot-air heating. In that case, take a look around your furnace. Remember, your system takes up air from around the furnace and blows it throughout your house! Repair any cracks in the foundation as they can lead to water seeping into the home.

- If you have a crawl space instead of a basement, this, too, must be investigated. Sometimes crawl spaces are even worse as they tend to be dark, wet, dirty, and moldy.

- If your home is built on a concrete slab, you may still have a problem. While this kind of construction avoids the problem of a wet basement, you could still have mold growing in the house. I remember one little boy who seemed to wheeze no matter what we tried. When I suggested replacing the carpeting, his mother discovered the carpeting was glued directly onto the concrete. She lifted the corner of the carpet and discovered that the entire floor of her child's bedroom was completely covered with mildew. They had to remove all of the carpeting, remove all mold, and have additional vapor-lock material placed under the new floor coverings.

- Molds love closets. Most closets are dark and, except in very dry climates, dank. Keep the door open and a lightbulb burning some of the time in the closet to help dry it out.

- Consider your indoor plants. Mold loves to grow in wet dirt. At a minimum, keep plants out of bedrooms.

- Beware of humidifiers or vaporizers. When a child develops a cough, many parents start running a vaporizer during the night. Not only are these devices largely ineffective at helping with the cough, but they also provide a great place for mold to grow. If you must use one of these gizmos, remember to dry out the reservoir that holds the water, including those hard-to-reach corners. Better yet, replace them periodically. (The small room-size ones aren't very expensive.) Humidification systems built into your heat system are also problematic. Often the ductwork is laid out so that water pools within the system. If there is standing water, there is mold. Incidentally, I think this is a very common problem in car air-conditioning systems. I frequently notice a slight mildew smell in cars, and I suspect mold is growing in the ventilation system. My sister Robin has major sneezing attacks when she is in her car. She's not allergic to the vehicle, she's allergic to mold within the ventilation system.

- Don't put away damp clothes or shoes. Hanging clothes outside to air them out will reduce mold. But this may also bring outdoor pollens indoors. I'm a great believer in tossing things into the dryer to be sure they're fully dry. Grass-filled sneakers or cleats can be left in the sun so that they can fully dry out.

- Clean kitchen and bathrooms with bleach solutions or other fungicides. Playing in the tub is lots of fun for young children, but mold is almost ubiquitous in bathrooms, so beware. An exhaust fan in the bathroom can be somewhat helpful, but, if possible, open a window.

- Discard moldy furnishings if possible. If you ever have a significant water leak, get rid of any carpeting or furniture that has remained wet long enough to develop mildew.

- Mold on the outside of the house can also be a problem. Window frames should be well sealed and any rotted shingles should be replaced. Mold loves to grow in rain gutters and downspouts, so clean them regularly. At least once a year, have old leaves cleaned out of the gutters and be sure that splash guards are designed to direct any water away from the house. In addition to helping with allergies and asthma, you'll extend the life of your home.

COCKROACHES

In recent years, we have discovered cockroaches are an important indoor allergen. Many people who live in city apartments must live in a constant state of war with these ubiquitous creatures, and at best can barely keep them at bay. To minimize cockroaches, eat only in the kitchen or dining room and don't let food be taken to the living room, den, or bedrooms. Use airtight containers for food; keep your kitchen and bathrooms really clean; wrap pipes with insulation to keep out roaches; use insecticides, bait, and traps. Remember to keep children out of your house until the smell completely subsides from insecticides.

MEASURES FOR REDUCING EXPOSURE TO COCKROACHES

- ■ Reduce the availability of food and crumbs.

- ■ Control dampness by preventing water leaks and using air-conditioning and dehumidifiers.

- ■ Restrict access by sealing around doors and caulking cracks in walls and floors.

- ■ Wage war with chemicals, bait, and traps.

PETS

As a dog lover myself, I understand how important pets are to families. Understandably, many parents feel that depriving their child of a dog or cat is a terrible thing. But it really doesn't make sense to have a cat if your child has to take four medications daily to counteract the allergic reaction. Cats are a particular problem, since they wipe their dander all over the furniture. And despite breeder claims, there really is no such thing as a nonallergenic dog.

But while I believe children really can have a perfectly happy childhood without a dog or cat, I have long since learned that parents "got to do what they got to do." So if pets are really important to you, turn to Chapter 9. This is so important that we are devoting a full chapter to it.

AVOIDANCE OF INDOOR POLLUTANTS

The list of indoor air pollutants is depressingly long. The list includes carbon monoxide, carbon dioxide, sulfur dioxide, nitric oxide, nitrogen oxides, formaldehyde, and all kinds of small, so-called respirable particles, otherwise known as soot. There is a clear relationship between particulate matter or soot in the air and increased heart and lung diseases.

- Open your windows whenever possible. I'm a big believer in fresh air. Over the last forty years our homes have become much better insulated and indoor air is not exchanged frequently.

- Do not smoke in the house. By far the most significant indoor pollutant is tobacco smoke. Although cigarette smoke is not an allergen per se, exposure to smoke in the home is a major cause of your children's sneezing and wheezing. Low-level cigarette smoke—not even enough to smell—can continuously irritate and inflame children's respiratory tracts, making them much more sensitive to allergens and infections. There have been numerous studies confirming that if an infant is exposed to very low levels, such as that on your clothing, they will then react worse next time they develop a cold (viral infection) or are exposed to an allergen. Believe it or not, many of the toxic substances in tobacco smoke are in higher concentrations in the plume of smoke drifting out of the end of a lit cigarette than in the smoke directly inhaled.

- Make proper maintenance of your heating and air-conditioning systems a priority.

- Make sure your furnace is ventilated to the outdoors.

- Make sure appliances have sufficient flues or ducts.

- Use glass doors on fireplaces to keep the smoke and soot from coming into the house. Parents frequently ask about fireplaces and wood-burning stoves. Open wood-burning fires put out a lot of particulate matter and perhaps even other toxic substances. If you really love a fireplace, try to install quality glass doors and keep them closed as much as possible. Keep in mind that fake logs and chemically treated kindling products may generate some really nasty fumes that no one should inhale. Wood-burning stoves are usually designed to supply heat, and they should be kept closed as much as possible.

- Be very careful with household cleaning products, polishes, and cooking oils. If you can smell it, it can bother your children. Potent cleaning sprays are really irritating to the respiratory tract of people with sensitive airways, so make sure the room is well ventilated and, if possible, keep your kids away until odors are gone. And covering up odors with other odor-producing products really makes very little sense from a pulmonary view-point. If you cook a lot, make sure you have a well-functioning hood with a fan over your range and use it.

MEASURES FOR REDUCING EXPOSURE TO INDOOR AIR POLLUTANTS

■ No tobacco smoke in your home.

■ On nice dry days, open your windows!

- Maintain your heating and air-conditioning systems properly and frequently.

- Keep fireplaces or wood-burning stoves closed or behind glass doors when possible.

- Ventilate your furnace and any gas appliances to the outdoors.

- Go easy on the household chemicals. If you can smell it, your child is breathing it.

AVOIDANCE OF OUTDOOR ALLERGENS

Outdoor allergens such as pollens and molds are difficult to control. I am very allergic to these kinds of things, and unfortunately, I have to close doors and windows and put on the air conditioner sometimes to avoid sneezing my brains out. Here are some things to consider:

- Pay attention to local pollen levels on TV, radio, newspapers, and the Internet.

- You'll often notice that after a rain the pollen count is lower, and when your area is overdue for rain, pollen counts will be high and allergy symptoms worse.

- Try to keep your child indoors when it's very windy, particularly between 6 A.M. and 10 A.M. the peak pollen hours. High winds can bring pollens from trees fairly far away.

- Use air-conditioning if possible, and make sure the air-conditioner filter is clean.

- On high pollen days, avoid using an attic fan or whole house fan, which brings in more pollen.

- Avoid drying clothes outside on the line on high-pollen days.

- Encourage your children to change their clothes after playing outside. Bathing or showering when they come in is also effective, because allergens are washed off.

WHAT ABOUT MOVING?

As I mentioned in Chapter 1, some families ask about the value of moving to another part of the country to improve allergies. Again, traveling sometimes temporarily helps but permanent moves probably won't make much difference because over time most people with allergies generally develop new allergies.

May and June are the worst months for my own hay fever. As it happens, almost every spring I travel for annual pulmonary research meetings held in a variety of different cities around the United States. If the conference is in a part of the country with a different pollinating season, I find that this five- to seven-day break from local tree and grass pollen helps me. Part of the benefit, however, probably comes from spending all day in air-conditioned conference rooms.

If your child is the type to develop allergies, sooner or later he or she will become allergic to the new list of pollens. Usually this takes about six months or so. Therefore, moving isn't the answer unless you plan to move every six months for the rest of your child's life.

Here are rough seasonal guides to ragweed, tree, and grass pollens. Needless to say, actual pollen counts vary significantly within these regions and there are many different species than those listed. And just as some days are worse than others, so are some seasons. Good luck.

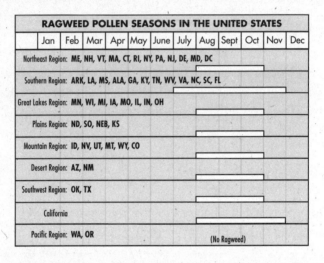

RAGWEED POLLEN SEASONS IN THE UNITED STATES	Jan	Feb	Mar	Apr	May	June	July	Aug	Sept	Oct	Nov	Dec
Northeast Region: ME, NH, VT, MA, CT, RI, NY, PA, NJ, DE, MD, DC												
Southern Region: ARK, LA, MS, ALA, GA, KY, TN, WV, VA, NC, SC, FL												
Great Lakes Region: MN, WI, MI, IA, MO, IL, IN, OH												
Plains Region: ND, SO, NEB, KS												
Mountain Region: ID, NV, UT, MT, WY, CO												
Desert Region: AZ, NM												
Southwest Region: OK, TX												
California												
Pacific Region: WA, OR								(No Ragweed)				

GRASS POLLEN SEASONS IN THE UNITED STATES	Jan	Feb	Mar	Apr	May	June	July	Aug	Sept	Oct	Nov	Dec
Northeast Region: ME, NH, VT, MA, CT, RI, NY, PA, NJ, DE, MD, DC												
Southern Region: ARK, LA, MS, ALA, GA, KY, TN, WV, VA, NC, SC, FL												
Great Lakes Region: MN, WI, MI, IA, MO, IL, IN, OH												
Plains Region: ND, SO, NEB, KS												
Mountain Region: ID, NV, UT, MT, WY, CO												
Desert Region: AZ, NM												
Southwest Region: OK, TX												
Pacific Region: WA, OR, CA												

Avoidance of Outdoor Air Pollutants

Symptoms of both allergies and asthma worsen as air quality worsens. Between soot (particulate matter) and smog (mostly car and truck exhaust), it is never a good sign when you can see air. Even before air can be seen, it fills up with all kinds of stuff that can bother your children. On the other hand, air

TREE POLLEN SEASONS IN THE UNITED STATES											
Jan	Feb	Mar	Apr	May	June	July	Aug	Sept	Oct	Nov	Dec

Northeast Region: ME, NH, VT, MA, CT, RI, NY, PA, NJ, DE, MD, DC
- Oak
- Pine
- Birch

Southern Region: ARK, LA, MS, ALA, GA, KY, TN, WV, VA, NC, SC, FL
- Oak
- Cedar
- Pecan

Great Lakes Region: MN, WI, MI, IA, MO, IL, IN, OH
- Oak
- Elm
- Maple

Plains Region: ND, SO, NEB, KS
- Oak
- Cedar
- Rye

Mountain Region: ID, NV, UT, MT, WY, CO
- Oak
- Cedar
- Maple

Desert Region: AZ, NM
- Oak
- Cedar
- Maple

Southwest Region: OK, TX
- Oak
- Cedar
- Elm

Pacific Region: WA, OR, CA
- Cedar
- Walnut
- Rye

pollution really doesn't explain the increased numbers of children who are bothered by asthma, since the incidence of asthma has been increasing even in areas with very clean air, and actually our overall air quality in the United States has improved, at least a bit, over the last twenty-five years. Nonetheless, if you or your child has any kind of respiratory condition, don't be shocked if you see more symptoms when pollution levels are high.

Information about air quality is easily available from local radio, TV, and Internet. If you hear that the quality is poor, avoid outdoor physical activity if it is not necessary. The key part of that sentence was "not necessary." Sports and other physical activities are very important parts of a child's life, and I certainly do not want to limit children from participating in activities they really enjoy. But during poor–air quality days, moderation and common sense are best.

TAKE-HOME MESSAGES

- If you suspect your child has an allergy to something, try to limit your child's exposure.

- While allergy-proofing an entire home can be daunting, at least reduce allergens in your child's bedroom. Decorate sparely and keep the number of stuffed animals to a minimum. Encase bedding in mite-proof covers and clean regularly.

- Keep your home dry enough to discourage mold, and if you use a vaporizer or humidifier during the winter, be certain to clean and dry it frequently.

- Open some windows when you can.

- Pay attention to seasonal warnings about allergy triggers such as ragweed, grasses, and pollen. They will remind you to pay attention to your child's medication levels, and there may be certain outdoor activities that you want to occasionally avoid.

NINE

The Truth About Cats, Dogs, Birds, and Other Animal Friends

Let me start by admitting up front that I'm a dog person, not a cat person. I hope you cat people out there will forgive me, but as I've mentioned before, I'm allergic to cats. Cats are beautiful, but I can't get near one without my eyes looking like Rosemary's baby's.

In our family, we've always had dogs. When I was young, a car hit our dog Taffy. My father rushed him to the animal hos-

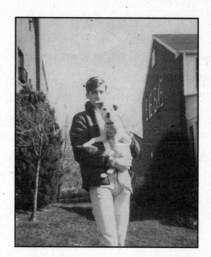

The author and Taffy, the amazing three-legged dog.

pital, and I really thought I would never see him again. As it happens, my dad was never the sort of person to fawn over a pet or have long conversations with one. Imagine my surprise a few hours later when he brought Taffy home with one leg gone. He lived many years after that, limping around on three legs, and very soon no one really seemed to notice Taffy's somewhat peculiar lurching motion.

Allergies to pets are very upsetting to kids but even more so for their parents. As you know, allergies can develop after years of exposure, long after a pet has become an irreplaceable member of your family. Although many allergists advise their patients to get rid of their pets, most people would rather suffer than part with a four-legged family member. After one study demonstrated the benefits of weekly cat shampoos to allergy sufferers, you could hear the whining and whimpering of half-drowned kittens all over the neighborhood. It seems that very few cats went along with that plan.

I mentioned Joe Weiker in Chapter 5, a patient's father who came to every visit with the predictable question: "Can we get a dog?" He felt that a dog was really important to overall child development and should be an essential part of his son Harold's life. As I said, I have a wonderful dog at home. But I know plenty of people who seem to grow up quite nicely without one, and I really don't think a family dog is as essential as, say, breathing. But Harold's dad felt strongly, and this was a problem, because Harold had really bad asthma. Within hours, he could go from feeling well to requiring a stay in the intensive care unit. And he definitely, absolutely, was allergic to dogs. When his dad first broached the subject, I expressed my concern, recited the risks involved, reassured him that the decision was his, and without really thinking about it, suggested that maybe he should get a turtle. I'm not sure why I said that. No special reason, the idea just popped into my head.

Next visit, sure enough, Dad waited until I was almost out the door and asked, "Are you sure we can't get a dog?" I sighed and again reviewed the situation. Kidding, I asked him once more to consider the turtle idea. He didn't seem appeased.

A couple of months later, I received a call from Harold's dad, who told me that he now agreed that a dog just wasn't a good idea. Apparently, he had decided to borrow a dog for the weekend. Within four hours of the dog's arrival, his son started to wheeze and had to go to the emergency room! So he called to thank me for the warning and to tell me they decided to buy a turtle after all. I congratulated him for making such a wise decision.

That wasn't the end of the story. Harold's dad called me a few weeks later, sounding very distraught, almost frantic. It seems that he did in fact buy his son a turtle, and sure enough, this turtle was a great pet—Harold really loved him. But there was one problem: The turtle never seemed to eat. Harold tried to interest him in all kinds of stuff, but nothing seemed right. So Harold and his dad brought the turtle to their local vet. The veterinarian hadn't seen one quite like this one, and he decided to get out his book and see if he couldn't figure out what kind of turtle he (or she) was. After leafing through this giant turtle book, the vet frowned and told Harold he thought the pet store had sold Harold's family an endangered species of turtle from South America. He called up a colleague from the Bronx Zoo, who explained that it was illegal for this turtle to remain a family pet and should be brought to the zoo immediately! Now Harold was very upset, and so was his dad.

Over the years I've been asked to write a lot of unusual letters for patients, but Harold's dad wins the prize. He asked me if I would write a letter explaining how important this turtle was to Harold's emotional development, and why it was really important that the turtle be permitted to stay with them. When I suggested that perhaps Harold could love another pet, his dad reminded me that the turtle was my idea in the first place. So, of course, I wrote the letter and the turtle stayed. Still has him, I think.

Key Point: *Animal sensitivity is one of the most frequent types of allergy, but a child who has these allergies almost always suffers from other types of allergies as well.*

What Causes Animal Allergies?

Any animal with fur or feathers can trigger an allergic reaction. The most likely culprits are proteins found in either saliva or dander (old shed skin cells) or in other pet secretions left all over the house. This protein is very tiny and can be inhaled not only into the nose, but also deep into the bronchial tubes, kicking off reactions that include sneezing and nasal congestion; red, itchy eyes; scratchy throats; or even coughing, wheezing, and difficulty breathing.

The Story on Dogs and Cats

Dogs shed a lot of this protein, but cats cause the most allergic reactions. Cats seem to be licking themselves constantly, spreading allergens from their saliva onto their fur. They also seem to secrete these allergy-causing proteins from sebaceous glands right onto their skin. They can rub this stuff all over sofas, chairs, wall treatments, carpeting, beds, curtains, drapes, etc. This stuff remains in your home, triggering reactions for months or years after a pet is gone!

Incidentally, male cats produce more of this cat allergen (known as Fel d 1) than female cats. Neutered male cats produce less allergen than fully grown male Toms. Studies suggest that dark and highly pigmented cats are more likely to cause allergic reactions than light-colored cats. By the way, dander and saliva are not the only sources of animal allergens. There have been some studies suggesting that urine from pets may also trigger allergic reactions.

Notice that when I described the makeup of animal allergens I didn't mention hair or fur. That's because they are not really the problem. Whether a dog sheds its fur, has hair, or is hairless doesn't really matter much, at least directly. That said, it is possible that some breeds of dog or cat are less likely to cause allergies than others. Some may produce less dander, and some lend themselves more easily to frequent shampooing. Now, I have to watch my words very carefully, because there is very little good scientific data to hang my hat on here. There are a lot of *claims* about hypoallergenic breeds, but I really am not able to substantiate these claims.

Key Point: *There is no such thing as a nonallergenic dog or cat.*

SOME DOG BREEDS THOUGHT TO BE HYPOALLERGENIC

American hairless terrier	Italian greyhound
Chinese crested	Kerry blue terrier
Peruvian Inca orchid	Maltese
Xoloitzcuintli (Mexican hairless)	Poodle
Basenji	Portuguese water dog

Bedlington terrier	Schnauzer
Bichon frise	Soft-coated wheaten terrier
Irish water spaniel	Tibetan terrier

I'm sure this list is incomplete. Likewise, some people believe that dogs prone to seborrhea (dry, scaly skin) will produce more dander and are therefore worse for allergy sufferers. While there may be some element of truth to this, keep in mind that highly allergic kids will react to the baldest, least flaky dog you can find.

SOME DOG BREEDS THOUGHT MORE LIKELY TO TRIGGER ALLERGIES

Cocker spaniel	Springer spaniel
West Highland white terrier	Chinese shar-pei
Basset hound	German shepherd
Irish setter	Afghan hound
Doberman pinscher	Dachshund

By the way, dog and cat hair can hold on to dust mites, molds, and pollens brought in from outdoors. So if your child is allergic to that other stuff, try not to let your pet run outdoors on a windy spring day and then proceed to rub all over the comforter on your child's bed.

Other Animals That Can Trigger Allergies

In addition to dogs and cats, kids can have allergic reactions to rabbits, horses, gerbils, mice, hamsters, ferrets, guinea pigs, and birds. Cows, pigs, and goats are also potential problems. There are even people who are allergic to ducks and geese. The most common offenders, besides dogs and cats, seem to be rabbits and horses. The droppings from birds, gerbils, mice, hamsters, and just about any other critter you can think of may also be a source of allergens. Not only can your child become allergic to that animal, but animal and bird droppings can also be a source for mold, dust, bacteria, and viruses, all of which can trigger reactions.

The other trigger from birds, of course, are feathers, which is why you should avoid feather comforters or pillows, or at least cover them with air-tight zippered encasings.

YOUR OWN CHILD'S SENSITIVITY

There are three factors that determine how badly a particular child reacts to a pet:

- How sensitive they are to that allergen. Some kids roll around on the carpet and just sneeze; others will turn into one big hive if they so much as let a cat or dog lick them.

- The "dose" of allergen. Some animals shed fewer allergens than others, and the number one determinant of that is animal size. The bigger the animal, the more they are likely to shed significant amounts of allergens. How a pet lives in your environment also matters. Cats seem to wipe their bodily fluids all over the upholstery, whereas dogs may actually stay off the couch if you make a point of it. Frequent washing of a pet can help, simply by lowering the dose to which you are exposed. I believe that many people seem to tolerate dogs that don't shed because dogs with "hair" (not fur) are always getting dirty and knotted, so many owners find themselves spending small fortunes on dog grooming and shampooing. While expensive and a pain in the neck, frequent washing and grooming does lower the allergen exposure.

- What other allergens are affecting your child. Your child's reaction to the same animal at different times can vary. If children are already sneezing and itching from other triggers, the animal may be the proverbial straw that breaks the camel's back. Allergy symptoms are cumulative. If you are already sensitized from pollens, dust, molds, or viral infections, the severity of a pet allergy may be accentuated.

Getting a Definitive Diagnosis

Diagnosis of other types of allergies is usually pretty straightforward. If your child repeatedly has symptoms soon after being exposed to something, they are probably allergic to that thing. However, pet owners often deny they are allergic to their dog or cat. There are three important reasons for this: First, people are usually exposed to their pet more or less every day, so it may be difficult to know for sure whether that animal is contributing to their problems. Second, remember that people who have allergies are almost never allergic just to the pet. So other triggers in their environment may confuse the issue. Third, pet owners often have very strong emotions about this issue, clouding their powers of detection.

Allergy tests may help, but remember they are just a guide. Theoretically, you could send your pet on vacation for a few weeks and see what happens. But allergens can really linger in a house, so it may take many repeated and meticulous cleanings to really get rid of pet allergens. Another option is to remove your child from the house, again for a few weeks. But since most kids also have other allergies, even this strategy can yield inexact results.

So What Would the Doctor Say?

There are two basic scenarios in my office: families who already have dogs or cats, and parents that are being begged for one by their children on a more or less daily basis. If families already have a pet, I don't automatically recommend they get rid of this important member of the family. If a young child is known to be allergic to that pet, finding a new home for their pet is an excellent choice, and some families are really just fine with that idea. (Although it seems to me not uncommon to find that one parent agrees with this idea, and the other parent is the one who has really bonded with the pet.) If parents really don't want to get rid of their pet, then there are some steps that can be taken to minimize a child's exposure.

When parents of young children ask me about adopting a pet, I try to gently discourage them if their child is already known to be allergic to other things or if they have significant asthma. Little kids spend a tremendous amount of time touching pets and lying on the floor, so their exposure will be much greater than that of older kids. I also urge parents to consider pets that don't have hair or fur, such as tropical fish or various reptiles. (If you do go the tropical fish route, remember that large aquariums increase the humidity, a great way to grow mold.)

There are some situations that would prompt me to recommend that a pet be removed. If your child has had a truly serious allergic reaction to a dog or cat, then I don't think you should take a chance. There is also a rare form of lung disease called hypersensitivity pneumonitis, in which patients experience a slow progression of fatigue, shortness of breath, and a general loss of energy. This can be caused by bird droppings and can result in permanent scarring of the lungs and permanent disability. In that case the bird must go.

If parents of an allergic child decide to adopt a pet anyway, I believe that overall, dogs are much less of a problem than cats. Bottom line: Cats are more allergenic, it is harder to keep them off the furniture or out of certain rooms, and it is much harder to shampoo them frequently.

I am perhaps somewhat biased because of my own cat allergy. We have these wonderful friends, the VanDeLays, who are generous hosts and love to entertain. They have often invited us to their beautiful home, and unfortunately, I find myself making excuses because of their cats. No matter how hard I try, no matter how many allergy pills I take before going, sooner or later my eyes turn itchy and red, my nose clogs up, the roof of my mouth begins to itch, and finally I am seized with repeated sneezing attacks. This is very embarrassing to me and everyone else, and it really is hard to continue normal conversation when I'm sneezing, blowing my nose, and wiping my eyes. The last time we went, I tried very hard not to sit on their sofas for long periods, finding all kinds of excuses for walking around, inspecting their books and CD collection, admiring drawings taped to the refrigerator, examining the paintings on the walls. All of that effort merely delayed the inevitable, and pretty soon I was thinking about walking outside to admire the outside of their house.

Imagine purposely bringing in an animal that may cause your child to feel the way I do at the VanDeLays. No matter how character building it is to have a pet, a child with strong allergies will enjoy it much less than a youngster who doesn't have to worry about sneezing, itching, or breaking out from exposure.

Getting a Dog

If your child has significant allergies or asthma, the best choice would be to not get a dog in the first place. But if you can't resist, then at least take care to minimize any risk.

If it is possible to buy your dog from a breeder you can visit their home with your child, and the breeder will likely allow your child to hug and kiss the dogs, rub his nose in their fur, even let the dog lick his skin. The most sensitive areas are on your child's neck and inside the arms. This is a way of testing your child's current level of allergic reaction to that particular breed. If you could borrow a dog of that breed for a few days, that would be great. Keep in mind that this doesn't mean your child won't develop an allergic reaction months or years later.

Lessening Allergic Reaction to Animals

Okay, you love your pet, but your child seems to be sneezing or wheezing, without any sign of a viral infection. What can you do?

- Minimize exposure to other allergens. Work to minimize any other allergens that you aren't quite so bonded with. In the previous chapter we reviewed steps that can be taken to minimize dust mites, mold spores, and pollens, as well as nonspecific irritants like cigarette smoke. Don't forget, symptoms of allergies are cumulative. If you really go on the warpath and minimize dust mites and mold spores, your children may better tolerate low doses of animal allergens. Since children with animal allergies almost always have other allergies, you won't see great benefit from losing your pet unless you also minimize other important allergens.

- Minimize exposure to animals other than your own. Avoid exposing your child to other pets. Does this make any sense? Actually it does. If your cat or dog offers a relatively low level of allergen exposure, your child may actually become quite used to it. But then if he's exposed to other pets and the total "dose" of allergen is increased, your child might develop symptoms not only triggered by his friend's dog but by the very pet he previously tolerated.

- Minimize the quantity of animal allergens in your home and car. Try to minimize reservoirs for animal allergens in your home. In other words, all of the same steps recommended for minimizing dust and dust mites also help with animal allergies. You know the stuff I'm talking about: Get rid of the carpets as much as possible. Avoid heavily upholstered furniture. Use blinds and shades that are easily dusted rather than heavy curtains. Buy those airtight covers for your mattresses and pillows. Make sure your vacuum cleaner isn't spreading more into the room than it sucks up. Animal allergens are very tiny and only very good vacuum cleaners will actually stop the stuff from getting sprayed right back into your room. Consider properly sized room air-cleaning systems with HEPA filters. Don't let anyone smoke in your home or car. On nice dry days, open some windows.

At a minimum, it seems reasonable to keep dogs or cats out of your children's bedrooms and certainly off their bed. It would also be nice if you could keep them off the furniture your kids use most, such as while they are watching TV. Try to encourage your children to wash their face, arms, and hands after playing with the pet. That sounds easy, doesn't it?

There are a variety of chemical products that you can spray on your upholstery or carpeting that purport to break down any allergens that are left after a good vacuum cleaning. I really don't know anything about them, but I imagine some of these can help lower the dose of allergen your child inhales. But instinctually, as a lung doctor, I really am not crazy about the idea of frequent spraying of chemicals in our homes. This just doesn't sit right with me. Our kids are already exposed to far more chemicals than previous generations, and I don't think we should add to this chemical burden without good evidence that the benefits outweigh the risks.

Indoor pets should be restricted to as few rooms in the home as possible. Isolating the pet to one room, however, will not limit the allergens to that room. Air currents from forced-air heating and air-conditioning may spread allergens through the house. If you do have forced-air heat or air-conditioning or are thinking of getting it, pay particular attention to filters or air cleaners in the system. Central-air cleaners can really help if they are regularly maintained.

- Make your pet as "hypoallergenic" as possible. Frequent washing and shampooing of dogs or cats lowers the allergen load, but it isn't certain how long this benefit lasts. If possible, shampooing your dog or any cat that thinks it's a dog once a week seems like a great idea. Shampooing your pet after they have hung out for a few days with other animals, such as in a kennel, can be very important. Dogs may come home covered in the dander of other dogs and even cats.

Some kids are sensitive to cat litter, especially brands with deodorizers. Try to avoid brands of litter that seem to generate a lot of dust, and make sure you or your kids pour litter into the pan very slowly to minimize any dust clouds. Some people even need to wear a face mask while they are changing the litter. If possible, don't place the litter box where air currents flow into the rest of the house. Probably this isn't the best chore for your allergic child.

MEASURES FOR REDUCING EXPOSURE TO ANIMAL ALLERGENS

- Keep pets off beds and preferably out of bedrooms completely.

- Avoid carpeting and upholstered furniture.

- Vacuum frequently with HEPA filters or at least double-thick bags.

- Use HEPA filters for bedrooms and main living rooms.

Allergy Shots for Animal Allergies

Allergy shots may help a child who is allergic, but remember that immunotherapy takes a long time to be effective, and during that time, minimizing environmental exposure is still very important. My impression is that immunotherapy works better for cats than for dogs. If your child is already reacting to the family dog on a daily basis, it may be difficult to desensitize him with shots. If your child is highly sensitive to start with, allergy shots are less likely to work.

Allergy Medications for Animal Allergies

The same medications discussed in detail in future chapters can help with pet allergies, so I am not going to discuss all of that now. Remember that these medications work much better if given before the exposure, rather than after the fact. And some, such as inhaled steroids for either asthma or nasal allergies, work best if you have been using them for at least a few days before the visit. Finally, my most important advice is to be prepared. If you are concerned about a trip to Grandma's house where there are two cats, make sure you bring a fresh supply of medications and work with your child's doctor to have a clear plan of what to do if your child begins to react.

I don't have any experience with either pet wipes or sprays for pets that reduce shedding. Two of the most popular brands, LoShed and Allerpet, apparently help decrease the frequency and severity of shedding in dogs, cats, and birds. While shedding is probably decreased, I am not sure how much difference they would make for someone who is highly allergic. The manufacturers claim these are very safe and helpful, though I know of no proof.

Vaccines for Pet Allergies

There is some exciting research going on with vaccines that may prevent cat allergies. Preliminary data has been encouraging, but this approach is still not ready for the marketplace. There are inevitably concerns about adding yet another vaccine to the long list of immunizations our children are already getting, and for the most part this one may not be truly necessary. Of course if your child wants to be a veterinarian, this approach may be a great advance.

Visiting Homes with Pets

This is a very tough issue. Over the years I have developed antennae for situations where I am getting caught between spouses, particularly ex-spouses. "Do you think it is okay for us to visit Grandma in North Carolina?" may sound like an innocent question but is actually a minefield. And of course the worst situation is when parents are divorced and one parent wants my opinion about Johnny spending the weekend with the other parent, who happens to have a cat or dog. Visits to friends are less likely to lead to protracted litigation, but are still problematic.

Remember, my basic philosophy is that I don't want children's allergies or asthma to affect their lifestyle. I have a very close family and I highly value family visits, so I usually recommend that you try to control your child's symptoms for important visits by utilizing appropriate premedication with antihistamines, nasal sprays, and asthma medicines. However, this does not always work, and honestly, with a highly allergic child, sometimes it is better to avoid some visits. This really has to be individualized and parents sometimes do have to make some tough decisions. Invite Jennifer's friends to your house rather than vice versa, for instance. If the annual visit to Granddad's house for Thanksgiving is really important and your child is clearly highly allergic, maybe you could gently suggest that Rover be removed a day or two before the visit and offer to pay for a really good cleaning before you arrive.

Pets: A Protective Factor?

What about the recently touted protective effect of having a dog or cat? You may have heard about some recent studies suggesting that there may be some long-term benefit from having a pet in your home. In one such study, about seven hundred kids were carefully followed from birth, and more than half of them had either a dog or cat in their home from the beginning. At six or seven years of age, the children who had been chronically exposed to pets were less likely to have significant pet allergy then the children who were raised in pet-free homes. This was pretty exciting news for animal lovers everywhere. In fact, there have now been a few studies suggesting that exposure to a dog in the first year of life may be protective to some children. But in my opinion, I really don't think you should let this information change your decisions about pets.

TAKE-HOME MESSAGES

- For the highly allergic child, it is best to avoid having a furry or feathered pet in the home. He can grow up to be a fine, well-adjusted adult without having a dog or cat.

- The child who is allergic to pets will be allergic to other things as well. Control of the other allergens may make a household pet more tolerable.

- There is no such thing as a truly nonallergenic cat or dog.

- When selecting a pet, take time to let your child visit the puppy (or a dog of the same breed) several times to see if there is a reaction.

- Ask your doctor about the possibility of immunotherapy and/or suitable medications.

- If your child is very allergic, you will need to be watchful about the presence of pets in the homes of friends and relatives. The severity of your child's reaction will dictate what steps are necessary.

TEN

Prevention and Management of Allergies and Asthma at School

Nicky is an adorable five-year-old, covered with freckles and full of energy. He's inquisitive, funny, and all smiles whenever he charges into my office. He and his mother recently visited me because Nick was about to start kindergarten. Though he was quite excited about the prospect, his mother, Cassandra, was scared stiff.

You see, I first met Nick and Cassandra two years ago in an emergency room. He had been flown to our medical center by helicopter after developing severe wheezing and hives after a snack was served at his preschool. After his second oatmeal cookie with peanuts, he sat down on the floor and started panting. By the time the local emergency medical team arrived, Nicky was turning blue and was in desperate need of help. As luck would have it, his mom had snuck away from her job for a few minutes to visit Nicky during snack time, so she was with him when he was whisked away by helicopter. Imagine what that experience must have been like for Nicky's mother! Is it any wonder she's afraid to let her baby go to school?

Parents have mixed emotions as their children become more independent. It's so exciting to watch their world open up, but the loss of control is equally frightening. Parents of children with allergies and asthma are in a particular quandary because they try so hard to protect them from allergic triggers and then send them to schools filled with allergic triggers.

From the class guinea pig and the dust mites, chalk dust, pollen, mold, or pet hair on another student's clothing to the spring flowers brought to the teacher by a well-meaning student, there are dozens of triggers in the classroom that may lead children with allergies to experience congestion, a runny nose, or itchy, watery eyes. Or in an asthmatic child, a full-scale response—coughing, wheezing, chest tightness—could be promoted. Symptoms can interfere with a student's participation in sports, school trips, physical education, and play activities as well as a child's energy level, concentration, peer relations, physical activities, and cognitive functioning.

"A lot of children just look glazed over when their allergies are bothering them," says a second-grade teacher. "Try as I might to reach them, the medicine or the allergic reaction just makes it really difficult for them to function during these times."

And if a child has food allergies, with the potential for very severe reactions and even anaphylaxis, parents can't help but be frightened. (Managing food allergies at school is addressed separately in Chapter 11.)

While we need to educate our children about possible risks, we don't want to paralyze them. We want them to love school, love new experiences, and feel confident and relaxed. Teaching our children to find the right balance between caution and adventure is tough, and no one expects you to get it just right all of the time. As in so many areas of parenting, no one can tell you the best approach. Let your instincts guide you.

What a Good School System Can Do to Help You

Filling out the health card for your child and sending it to the school nurse is just the beginning of what you need to do to be certain your child is well cared for at school. If you have a child with serious allergies or asthma, meet with his or her classroom teacher or counselor at the beginning of the year and inform him or her about your child's situation. See the Appendix for a sample of what the Asthma and Allergy Foundation of America (AAFA) recommends your teacher have as part of the classroom record on your child. For most families, this initial meeting will be all that is necessary. From there a good school system will put the following in motion:

- Schools must know their legal responsibilities, including that children cannot be excluded from school activities solely based on food allergies. Federal laws designed to protect students with food allergies include the Rehabilitation Act of 1973, section 504; Individuals with Disabilities Education Act (IDEA); and Americans with Disabilities Act of 1990 (ADA).

- Schools should identify a core team, usually including the school nurse, teacher, principal, and food service manager or director, who will work with you to establish a good plan.

- All school personnel who interact with the student on a regular basis should understand food allergy, recognize the symptoms, and know what to do in an emergency.

- Staff who know how to inject epinephrine (EpiPen) should be in school. In one study it was found that only about 35 percent of schools had anyone who knew how to correctly administer the medication. For that matter, only 25 to 30 percent of doctors and doctors in training knew how to use the medication themselves.

- Schools need to look carefully at their policies about carrying medications. Ideally a child who previously has had a significant reaction to foods should be permitted to carry an EpiPen with him. As you know, this is the lifesaving medication epinephrine prepackaged in a syringe with a needle, ready for use. Supply your child with a safe carrying case for this purpose.

- When a child with known food allergies is identified, the health team at school should develop an individual health plan (IHP) for the student, focusing on the following:
    * Medical documentation and emergency action plans
    * Staff training, including special teachers, substitute teachers, maintenance, and housekeeping personnel
    * Education programs for all children in the classroom and school
    * Cafeteria and playground issues
    * Assemblies, field days, field trips, and bus transportation

If you feel that asthma and allergy triggers in school are not getting appropriate attention, become more active. Remember that if your child is bothered by something, so are many others, so speak to other parents. Speak to your local PTA and school board. Your children are going to be in school for many hours each day for many years. Lots of class pets have been moved out of classrooms where children are allergic; many cafeterias have peanut-free tables; and some school districts have parent committees to deal with environmental issues such as air quality in the schools. Things can happen when parents become active.

Environmental Allergens

Scant attention is usually paid to air quality in schools and day care centers until a crisis occurs. Indoor air quality is a problem in more than 50 percent of the nation's schools. General maintenance is very important in creating a healthy indoor environment. Three of the major contributors to indoor air pollution are heating and ventilation systems, leaky pipes, and carpeting. Leaky roofs and pipes and inadequately sealed windows let moisture build up, and wherever there is dampness there is mold. School carpets are a fertile environment for growing organisms that can trigger allergies and asthma. If a carpet gets wet, it must be thoroughly dried within twenty-four hours to prevent mold from forming.

Some schools form environmental committees to assess and prioritize what needs to be done, and a few districts hire environmental service companies to help assess the indoor air quality of a school. Each parent can help in this effort. (Check with the Environmental Protection Agency for additional information.)

Mold Is a Serious Problem in Schools

In my experience mold is the biggest allergy problem in most schools. The mold found in a school environment is generally a potent trigger of allergies and asthma; however, your child is unlikely to encounter what the popular press has publicized as "toxic" mold, which can be fatal, especially for infants and young children. This type of mold was reported in the press to cause serious respiratory disease in young infants, but it appears to be very unusual.

Molds can be hidden under rugs, behind wallpaper, and anytime a school plumber hasn't had time to come by to fix a drip or a leak. Portable classrooms are also breeding grounds for mold. If you want to grow mold, here's the recipe: Pour concrete directly onto the ground and glue carpeting on it. Cover with a poorly constructed shack and wait until the rainy season.

Key Point: *Mold usually grows in moisture. It is essential to control any water leaks.*

The Environmental Protection Agency (EPA) has published excellent recommendations on their web site (*http://www.epa.gov/iaq/molds/index.html*) for how schools and commercial buildings can prevent mold growth. The following are good to keep in mind:

- Signs of water damage (damp carpet, stained ceiling tiles) or a general feeling of dampness in school should raise suspicion about the presence of mold. Ask if the source of the dampness can be investigated, and anything that doesn't dry out well (such as carpet) should be removed.

- Anything that becomes moldy should be removed from the classroom. Throw out old newspapers and check bookshelves for signs of mold. If growing mold is a classroom science project, can it be done in the winter when other allergy triggers are less likely to be present?

Little Steps Can Help

Here are some things to notice as you visit school. Some may be serious enough to bring to the attention of school administration; others you may want to discuss with the classroom teacher. You may want to photocopy this list and give it to appropriate school personnel.

WHAT SCHOOLS CAN DO TO CREATE A HEALTHIER ENVIRONMENT

- Air-conditioning and heating-system vents should be cleaned periodically, particularly after any construction projects. While fresh air is always desirable, trees, shrubs, and flowers should be trimmed back from the windows.

- Review what is in the classroom. Anything old that is a dust catcher or may have developed mold should be cleaned thoroughly or discarded.

- General cleanliness is important. No food should be kept in the classroom, and the room should be kept free of scented cleansers or disinfectants. Spills should be cleaned up immediately (rugs require immediate cleaning and drying). The classroom should be dusted and vacuumed regularly, and all trash should be removed. Vacuuming and cleaning with chemical substances should be done after school hours.

- Classrooms for preschoolers or early elementary school children should have allergen-proof pillows and washable mats, rather than rugs, if they nap at school. Avoid feather filling.

- Before a pet is added to the classroom, check with families of students to be certain there are no known allergies to pets. Some districts are writing policies against fur-bearing animals in the classroom, and the EPA has suggested that alternatives to animals be used when possible.

- If a pet is in the classroom, keep it in its cage as much as possible, and keep the cage away from the ventilation system to prevent circulating allergens through the room or the building. Children who may be sensitive to dander should be seated in another part of the classroom.

- Plants can trigger allergic reactions. Plants in projects have a purpose, but may not be necessary as extraneous decoration. Consider other ways to brighten and warm the room.

- Science experiments should be done in a well-ventilated room using an exhaust system, and care should be taken with all dangerous supplies. Even a basic scientific necessity like formaldehyde (for dissection in biology) can be an irritant. Some school systems now study "microchemistry" instead of chemistry, improving the situation for students with allergies or asthma since smaller quantities mean less potency. Asthma sufferers may require special masks for labs such as chemistry labs where odors are strong.

Key Point: *Minimizing exposure to environmen-*
tal allergens is not your child's prob-
lem, it's the school's problem.
Sometimes parents have to get
involved and remind schools of that.

Animals in the Classroom

The subject of animals in the classroom—or the lack thereof—tends to be a highly charged issue. I know that many well-meaning teachers feel that having furry little friends in the classroom is of great educational benefit and is also a lot of fun for the kids. But for children who are allergic, they present a major problem. Rabbits, hamsters, and guinea pigs shouldn't live in the classroom, and visits from cats and dogs should occur only if no one in the classroom is allergic. If anyone is going to suffer from the visit, it just isn't worth it.

If your child has an allergy to animals, make sure teachers know this. If your child is old enough to understand why they should avoid kissing and touching animals that they are allergic to, explain it to them carefully and repeatedly so that if there is a class pet, your child is conditioned to avoid exposure to the greatest extent possible.

If your child's allergies or asthma seem to be triggered by something in the classroom and you haven't uncovered anything, don't discount animals. Some children are so allergic they react to dog hair on someone else's backpack or cat hair that clings to the clothing of a teacher. Avoidance of these types of exposures is difficult, but there may be solutions: Can coats and backpacks be stored outside the classroom? Could your child share a cubby with a child who does not have a pet at home? One child with a cat allergy found that what seemed to be an allergy to the teacher was actually an allergy to her clothing—she had five cats at home. Fortunately, the discovery was made early, and before the child had really settled in he was transferred to a different classroom.

Field Trips

Schools are generally well prepared to travel safely with large groups of students. In some districts, health information on all children with any health issues is pulled and all necessary medication is taken along. Teachers are loaded with instructions and medicines for the children with asthma, the ones with allergies to bee stings or shellfish, as well as all other issues affecting school-age children. (Antidepressant medications, ADHD treatments, and insulin are just a few of the other medications that are taken along.) Inquire what the procedure is in your district. If the teachers don't automatically take along this medical information and your child has a potentially serious condition, talk to the teacher and be sure that adequate steps are taken to safeguard your child's safety on field trips. Field trips are a source of understandable anxiety for parents. EpiPens should always be brought along, and someone on the trip should know how to use them. There should also be a clear plan for emergencies.

Management of Exercise-Induced Asthma in School

Recognition and control of exercise-induced asthma is so important, Chapter 16 is completely devoted to this topic. But there are some major points worth emphasizing here:

1. Exercise-induced bronchospasm is much more common than most people think. For some kids, this may be their only sign of asthma.
2. If kids seem to be breathing fast or tiring easily in

gym class, the least likely explanation is that they are lazy or poorly motivated.

3. Exercise-induced bronchospasm can be controlled. Don't settle.

4. If medications are needed to prevent exercise-induced bronchospasm, see if it can't be controlled with medication given before school, so as not to interrupt your child's day.

5. Even recess can trigger asthma. Sitting still in class can be tough, and some kids like to run around like maniacs when they have the opportunity. We must do everything we can to allow them to run as fast as they wish.

The Older Child: Taking Responsibility

If your child is old enough, help him understand the allergens that trigger reactions. Talk to your child about the need to take symptoms in stride and do something about them. Children need to understand it is important to respond to asthma symptoms immediately and not ignore warning signs that may progress to a full-blown asthma attack. The best management of asthma and allergies involves a long-term commitment to taking appropriate medications, so it's important to stress to your child that medical recommendations should be followed carefully.

Many schools insist that students' personal medications be kept in the health office. While this may be necessary with younger children who will need help in taking medication or using an inhaler, this is problematic with older children. Some medications are best taken when symptoms first appear. The child in class without medication must first find an appropriate time to ask the teacher if he can be excused from the classroom, and then he needs to get to the health office quickly. In addition to being inconvenient, this procedure makes it a big deal to go and take medication, and adolescents are particularly resistant to anything that makes them different.

Because asthma sufferers can have sudden and serious attacks, mature children (so deemed by parents and physician) should be given permission to carry inhaled medications in their backpacks. Find out if your child's school permits children to keep inhaled medications in their possession. For those old enough to know how to handle medications, the best management of the disease involves having the inhalers in their possession, as well as an appropriate spacer or holding chamber.

If your child still seems to be having difficulty with learning, alertness, or endurance, ask your physician if any medications should be adjusted.

School Checkup: A Periodic Review List

1. How is your school's air quality? Does it seem like there is a problem?
2. Do they try to minimize pets with fur or feathers, dust in carpets or upholstery, cockroaches, or fumes or odors from cleaning chemicals, paint, perfumes, or pesticides?
3. Are there any water leaks in the classrooms? Do you smell mildew anywhere? If so, that means there are mold spores. Are they planning to stop those leaks?
4. Does your school have a full-time nurse on the premises? If not, do they at least have a nurse available to help guide them in the care of students with asthma and allergies?

5. Does your school offer educational programs for their staff about allergies and asthma?

6. Are mature children with asthma permitted to carry their own medications?

7. Is it easy for children to be able to take prescribed medicines during school hours with minimal disruption of their day?

8. Does your school have a clear plan to manage a child with a severe allergic reaction or asthma attack?

9. Are children with asthma encouraged to take their inhalers if needed before gym and recess?

10. Will your school's physical education staff permit children to choose modified or alternative exercise programs when medically necessary?

TAKE-HOME MESSAGES

- Set up a meeting with your child's teacher or counselor to discuss your child's allergies or asthma. Schools are prepared to handle almost anything if they are informed.

- Become active in school committees that concern anything from lunchroom to environmental issues. The situation for children with allergies and asthma has improved markedly in a short time, largely because of parents helping to build awareness.

- Be certain your school has the medications your child might need in case of an emergency. Send in new supplies annually so that medicines aren't out of date.

- Older children need to take responsibility for their own health, so make sure they understand allergy or asthma triggers and can try to avoid them. If possible, work with your child to take responsibility for carrying and taking his own medicine.

ELEVEN

Preventing Allergic Reactions to Foods

You've been reading a lot about preventing exposure to potential allergens, and nowhere is this more important than with food allergies. One family I know has to prepare—at home—everything their five-year-old son eats so that they can control the substances he's exposed to; another mom calls to check on the menu with all party hosts whenever her daughter is invited somewhere. If there's something to which her daughter is allergic, a separate meal or piece of cake will accompany her daughter to the party. Another mother remarked of her nervousness as her ten-year-old with severe food allergies started a new summer program: "This will be the first time in her life that she's eaten food that I haven't prepared or checked for her."

While a child who is allergic to pollen can take an antihistamine to minimize his symptoms, the child with food allergies has little recourse, and unsuccessful avoidance can be life-threatening. For this reason, it's important to do what you can to reduce the likelihood of your child encountering the food that triggers an allergic reaction.

Schools must pay attention to children with severe food allergies. It is hard to keep children with peanut allergies from touching a bit of peanut butter smeared on the lunch table or trading for a bite of something that may have been prepared using peanut oil, so parents must work to help schools manage this issue.

Almost all children who develop severe allergic reactions to foods also have asthma, and reactions to food will be worse if their asthma is poorly controlled (see Chapter 13).

Key Point: *If your child has had a severe*
food allergy, you should obtain
a medical alert bracelet or
necklace that states the specific
allergy in case you are not there.

Handling a Severe Reaction

Anaphylactic reactions are life-threatening, and we have devoted a separate chapter to the subject (Chapter 20), but if you feel your child is having a severe reaction, act quickly:

- Seek medical attention by calling 911 or the operator (0) or go to an emergency room.

- Administer epinephrine (adrenaline). If you don't have an EpiPen, ask the emergency medical technicians for one.

- Even if you've administered the EpiPen, you still must take your child to an emergency room. Once the medication wears off, the reaction may return.

- It is far better to call 911 or go to an emergency room and be embarrassed if no reaction occurs than to ignore the early signs of allergic reactions and not get help in time.

Treatment of Food Allergies

As described in Chapter 6, offending foods must be accurately identified and you need to eliminate that food or related food substance from your child's diet. This means reading detailed ingredient lists, often in very small print, must be a part of your life. Food labeling has gotten better over the years (more complete and sometimes in larger type), but there is room for improvement. The allergy community (patients, their families, and physicians) must continue to press their case for making labels less confusing and easier to read.

There are, of course, many medications reviewed throughout this book that can help relieve symptoms of food allergies: antihistamines for itching, inhalers for asthma, etc. Sometimes parents ask me if giving their child a medication prior to possible exposure to a known food allergen will stop the reaction. This doesn't work.

Some people have tried allergy shots for food allergies. Unfortunately, the benefits of this approach have never been proven and I really can't recommend them. Someone once suggested that if you place a diluted solution of a particular food under your child's tongue about thirty minutes before he eats that food, you could avoid an allergic reaction. Sorry, I don't believe this works and in fact, it can be very dangerous.

Hope in the New Anti-IgE Therapy?

As I mentioned in Chapter 7, a new form of therapy involving regular injections of anti-IgE is now on the market. Children known to be highly allergic to nuts may be able to tolerate eating at least some nuts after receiving this therapy. This may prove to be a real gift for such children and their understandably anxious parents. However, we do not yet know about the long-term risks or benefits of this new approach.

> **Key Point:** *You should have epinephrine (adrenaline) available for your child at home, at school, and wherever your child is going to be. Keep track of expiration dates.*

How to Help Your Child Avoid Specific Foods

Here are recommendations for avoiding the most common food allergens: milk, soy, wheat, shellfish (shrimp, crayfish, lobster, and crab), peanuts, tree nuts (such as walnuts), fish, and eggs.

TIPS FOR PREVENTING ALLERGIC REACTIONS TO COW'S MILK

- Many people rely on kosher symbols on products to determine if a product is milk-free. There are two symbols that can be helpful: a D for the word "dairy" next to K or U indicates the product contains milk protein. A DE indicates that the equipment used was shared with dairy (milk). A product marked "Parev" or "Parve" contains neither meat nor dairy. However, while these are considered milk-free according to religious specifications, there still may be very small amounts of milk, enough to trigger a reaction in someone highly sensitive.

- Many nondairy products contain casein, which is one of the milk proteins that can cause allergic reactions. Canned tuna fish is one such product. Even some meat may contain casein as a binder. Check ingredients carefully.

- Goat's milk is not a safe alternative to cow's milk. Their proteins are very similar.

- There are a variety of ingredients that sound like they are related to milk but actually aren't: cocoa butter, cream of tartar, calcium lactate, calcium stearoyl lactylate, sodium lactate, and sodium stearoyl lactylate.

- Sometimes you can substitute water or fruit juice for milk in baking or cooking. There are also whole cookbooks dedicated to milk-free cooking.

- Beware of deli meat slicers that may be used for both meat and cheese.

- Many restaurants use butter on steaks after they have been grilled, and the butter won't be visible after it melts.

Tips for Preventing Allergic Reactions to Eggs

- Some brands of egg substitutes actually contain egg whites.

- Some packaged cooked pastas may contain egg or were processed on equipment shared with egg-containing pastas. Boxed, dry pastas and fresh pastas are usually egg-free.

- If your child is allergic to eggs, flu shots are usually not recommended, since the influenza vaccines are grown in egg embryos. Actually, there is very little egg protein and reactions even in people with known egg allergy are quite rare. But it is probably best avoided unless your child is at high risk for complications from influenza.

- MMR vaccine (measles, mumps, and rubella) is recommended for children who are allergic to eggs. The risk of reaction is very small and the benefits are great.

- For some recipes that call for eggs, other ingredients can be substituted:
  * 1 tsp. yeast, dissolved in ¼ cup warm water
  * 1 packet of gelatin, mixed just before using, with 2 tbsp. warm water
  * 1 tsp. baking powder mixed with 1 tbsp. water and 1 tbsp. vinegar

- Beware of foam or milk toppings on fancy coffee drinks, eggs are sometimes included.

TIPS FOR PREVENTING ALLERGIC REACTIONS TO PEANUTS

- If your child is allergic to peanuts, they should avoid eating any chocolate candies unless they are absolutely certain there is no risk of contamination during manufacturing procedures. This is a really big problem for a lot of kids.

- Artificial nuts are sometimes peanuts that have been deflavored and then reflavored, so don't take a chance on them.

- Most allergists recommend that peanut-allergic patients are better off avoiding any kind of nuts, such as tree nuts, even if testing was negative to these.

- Some people have substituted other types of nut butters, such as cashew nut butter, for peanut butter. Again the problem is that some nut butters are produced on equipment used to process peanut butter, placing your child at risk.

- Foods sold in bakeries and ice cream shops may have come in contact with peanuts.

- Peanut-allergic children can eat sunflower seeds, but these are best avoided since they are often processed on the same equipment used for processing peanuts.

- Mandelonas are peanuts soaked in almond flavoring.

- Arachis oil is peanut oil, so don't be deceived.

- Certain types of cuisine use peanuts quite heavily, including Chinese, Vietnamese, Thai, Korean, Indonesian, and some African styles. Even if the particular dish you ordered is free of peanuts, cooking pans, woks, and utensils may be contaminated. So I'm afraid I can't recommend that a child with known peanut allergy take a chance and go to these restaurants.

- Actually, most people who are allergic to peanuts can tolerate peanut oil. However, if the peanut oil has been contaminated with peanuts during processing, you could have a problem.

- Some kids grow out of peanut allergy, but this must be carefully proven. After about five years of no reactions, most allergists will first obtain a blood test looking for very low, specific peanut IgE levels, followed by a challenge with a small amount of peanut in a controlled setting.

- If your child with peanut allergy has a twin, that twin is also at high risk for peanut allergy. In one study, 65 percent of identical twins and 7 percent of fraternal twins also showed signs of peanut allergy.

- While there are reports of children who have allergic reactions just from sitting at a lunch table with kids eating peanut butter, this is rare. If your child has had a significant reaction to peanuts, ask your allergist about this. Unfortunately, I know of no completely accurate way to predict this kind of thing. That's why you have to be certain the school is prepared.

TIPS FOR PREVENTING ALLERGIC REACTIONS TO TREE NUTS (E.G., CASHEWS, ALMONDS, PECANS, AND WALNUTS)

- Many different foods frequently contain tree nuts, including cereals, ice cream, barbecue sauces, and crackers.

- Artificial and natural flavorings in processed foods may contain tree nuts.

- Mortadella may contain pistachios.

- Most people who are allergic to tree nuts tolerate coconut, which is actually the seed of a fruit tree. However, there are occasionally people who have reacted to coconuts.

- Most allergists will recommend that if your child is allergic to one type of tree nut, they should avoid all tree nuts, since she could develop allergic reactions to other tree nuts.

- Nutmeg is safe for people allergic to tree nuts. Nutmeg is derived from the seeds of the tropical tree *Myristica fragrans*.

TIPS FOR PREVENTING ALLERGIC REACTIONS TO FISH OR SHELLFISH

- Allergists generally recommend that if your child has had an allergic reaction to one type of fish, or has even had a positive skin test to one fish, they should avoid all species of fish, including shellfish—shrimp, crab, lobster, and crayfish.

- Fish proteins can actually become airborne during cooking and cause an allergic reaction.

- There have been reports of people having reactions just walking through a fish market.

- If your child is allergic to fish or shellfish, you should avoid fish or seafood restaurants altogether. Although these restaurants often offer a "nonfish entrée," the kitchen areas where these foods are being prepared might very well be contaminated with fish protein.

- Carrageenan, or Irish moss, is not a fish. This product is used in all kinds of foods, including dairy foods, and does not have to be avoided by people allergic to fish or shellfish.

- Remember that Caesar salad dressings and some steak sauces contain anchovies. Anchovies are also sometimes in caponata, a traditional Sicilian relish.

- If you have a specific fish allergy but really want to have some fish in your diet, ask your allergist about the possibility of being challenged with other types of fish.

- People with fish or shellfish allergies do not have to be particularly concerned about reactions to the contrast materials most often used in X-ray procedures. There is no particular cross reaction between fish and these iodine-containing materials. There has been an erroneous belief that people who are allergic to fish, especially shellfish, are actually allergic to the iodine contained in these fish. This is not true—the allergy is to various proteins in the fish.

TIPS FOR PREVENTING ALLERGIC REACTIONS TO SOY

- Soybeans and soy products are often found in soups, cereals, crackers, baked goods, canned tuna, sauces, some peanut butters, and of course certain infant formulas.

- Although soy is not a major part of an American diet, soybeans have found their way into so many different kinds of food products that eliminating all of those foods can result in a very unbalanced diet. Consult a dietician to make sure your child is still receiving adequate nutrition.

- Most people who are allergic to soy can usually tolerate soybean oil and soy lecithin.

TIPS FOR PREVENTING ALLERGIC REACTIONS TO WHEAT

- It is important to distinguish between a true allergic reaction to wheat, which many kids outgrow, and celiac disease, which is a lifelong sensitivity to a chemical in wheat called gluten.

- If you like to bake, it is possible to substitute other types of flour such as rice flour, potato starch flour, soy flour, and corn flour for wheat flour.

- Once again, some surprising foods contain wheat, including some brands of ice cream and hot dogs. Some types of imitation crabmeat also contain wheat.

- In some Asian dishes, wheat flour is sometimes shaped and flavored to look like shrimp, pork, or beef.

- Kamut is a cereal grain related to wheat.

- Spelt is a type of wheat and not safe for wheat-allergic people.

The Challenge of Cross-Reactivity and the Oral-Allergy Syndrome

If your child has had an allergic reaction to a food, your doctor will counsel avoidance of similar foods that may also cause this reaction. For instance, if your child is allergic to shrimp, she probably needs to stay away from crab, crayfish, and lobster.

There are also less obvious kinds of cross-reactivity that can baffle parents and doctors. One of the most common inhaled allergens in the United States is ragweed, which pollinates in the fall. During that season, when some kids are highly sensitized to ragweed, they may also itch or have other allergic symptoms when they eat bananas, cantaloupe, or other melons.

This is an example of the so-called oral-allergy syndrome. Kids with this syndrome first become allergic to pollens, and then they become sensitive to similar proteins in foods, with symptoms such as itching, redness, and swelling around the mouth. Another example of cross-reactivity occurs in people who are highly allergic to birch tree pollen, a spring allergen. During the tree pollen season, some people will find they also have allergic reactions to apples, pears, peaches, potatoes, carrots, almonds, and hazelnuts. Children allergic to grass pollen may react to tomatoes. These allergy-producing proteins tend to be in higher concentrations in the peel of some fruits. Allergic reactions may not occur except during and soon after the pollinating season, further confusing the diagnosis. Fortunately, most of the time, these allergic reactions remain localized to the area around the mouth, though occasionally they can progress into more severe reactions.

Managing Food Allergies in School

Keeping children with food allergies safe requires teamwork with families, school personnel, and the kids themselves. This is a big responsibility and it's not always easy. Parents must take the lead in what needs to be done to safeguard their child. There are some specific responsibilities that can only be shouldered by the family.

FAMILY RESPONSIBILITIES

- Notify the school of your child's particular food allergies, and work with the school team to develop a plan that includes the classroom, the cafeteria, the school bus, school-sponsored activities, and after-care programs.

- Give the school a written food allergy action plan, which includes instructions and medications as directed by a physician (see page 194).

- Educate your older child in the self-management of her food allergies, how to read food labels, strategies to avoid unsafe foods, and how and when to tell an adult she may be having an allergic reaction.

- Reinforce with your own child why she shouldn't eat other children's food or snacks, no matter how tempting. Children do not usually feel comfortable asking what the ingredients are in their friend's lunch bags, and I wouldn't trust word-of-mouth information anyway.

- Pack extra snacks for special occasions in your child's class when you know she won't be able to eat the same as the rest of the class. Stress that she should tell you when she gets tired of what you send for these occasions, and assure her that you won't be insulted or upset.

- Don't be embarrassed to spread the word among parents of the rest of the class about the presence of a child with significant food allergies. If there is a child with peanut allergy, a teacher will usually send home a notice asking parents not to send in snacks with peanuts in them. The other kids can live without peanuts at school.

- Remember to replace medications including EpiPens after use or upon expiration.

Key Point: *Supply your child's school with at least two EpiPens. At the start of every school year make sure that they are not expired or will not expire during that year.*

SNACK TIME

Make sure there is control over snacks that come into the classroom. This is particularly important if your child is allergic to peanuts or tree nuts because nuts are frequently found in many of the popular snacks kids bring to school.

One way to establish a "safe snack" program is to ask all parents to contribute to a fund from which all snacks and birthday treats are purchased. The parent of a child with food allergies can make all of the purchases from this snack fund, taking note of all ingredients. While this is a bit of a hassle for you, the parent, the method permits you to breathe easy knowing that the foods served are all on the "approved" list. Another option is for the parent of the food-allergic child to supply a list of safe snacks, and all parents then agree to send in only snacks on that list.

Some schools have agreed to designate certain classrooms as free of the specific allergen of concern, e.g., "nut-free." That way anyone who comes into the classroom, such as art and music teachers or substitute teachers, are warned not to bring anything in that may contain nuts. It is also a good idea to ask all students and teachers to wash their hands on entering the room at the start of the day and after returning from recess.

IN THE CAFETERIA

Some schools designate certain tables as peanut or allergen-free. Don't let the school forget about the social aspects of such a plan. Your child with peanut allergy should not feel isolated. If such tables are established, all classmates should rotate to these tables, and of course bring in safe snacks if they are to sit at that table. After lunch, those tables can be washed carefully and put away so they are not used for other projects during the school day or after school hours that may introduce allergens.

Cafeteria and food services staff members need to be included in any educational programs. The United States Department of Agriculture has developed guidelines for food service staff as part of their child nutrition program (*www.fns.usda.gov*).

Lunchroom personnel (cafeteria workers, teachers' aides, supervising teachers) should know about all food allergies. A complete list of a child's food allergies should be provided. If staff will have access to epinephrine for treating your child in case of an attack, provide an identification sheet with the child's name, photo (since lunchroom personnel don't always know a child by name), and specific allergy for distribution to appropriate personnel. Lunchroom supervisors should be trained to administer epinephrine in case of an emergency. With the onset of anaphylactic shock, there is little time to look for the school nurse.

An identification card on each child with food allergies should be kept in the lunchroom (see below).

```
┌─────────────────────────────────────────────┬──────────────┐
│                                              │              │
│   Name of Child                              │              │
│   _____           │              │
│                                              │              │
│   Allergy                                    │              │
│                                              │              │
│   _____           │              │
│                                              │              │
│   Appropriate treatment                      │              │
│   _____           │              │
│                                              │              │
└─────────────────────────────────────────────┴──────────────┘
```

Parents should also work with schools to establish a no-food-trading policy and to stress the importance of not permitting food into the classroom.

Parents and teachers who aren't directly affected by these issues sometimes can be very thoughtless. Nothing upsets me more then when I hear that parents of children with food allergies are sometimes made to feel overly neurotic.

Key Point: *It's your child. Don't ever apologize for worrying too much.*

TAKE-HOME MESSAGES

- Food allergies are rare but can be life-threatening. Parents of children with food allergies need to work very hard on avoidance of this particular type of allergen.

- Obtain a medical alert bracelet for your child that specifies the food to which she is allergic.

- Get a prescription for epinephrine, also known as adrenaline (usually an EpiPen), from your doctor; learn how and when to administer it.

- Make it a habit to read food labels. You'll also find yourself quizzing restaurant staff and people who host your child for a meal about the items on the menu.

- You may need to send food along with your child instead of letting him eat what will be provided.

- Meet with your child's teacher, counselor, or school nurse about your child's food allergy.

- Schools should have an emergency plan for the cafeteria, and the staff members who supervise lunchtime should be prepared to implement it.

- Depending on the severity of your child's food allergies, you may need to establish a "safe snack" program for the classroom.

- Many parents always send extra food with their child in case they encounter food on a play date that they can't eat.

- Children need to learn from an early age about their food allergy. They need to know not to trade food at lunch or snack time and learn when to be wary of certain foods.

- If your child has a severe allergy to food, never be embarrassed by your hypervigilance. You really have no choice.

TWELVE

Prevention and Management Away from Home: Sleepovers, Summer Camp, Family Trips, Scuba Diving, and Mountain Climbing

I once got a call from the father of Erin, a teenage patient of mine, asking me if it was okay for his daughter to climb Mount Rainier. (Keep in mind that my general philosophy is that all kids should be able to do almost anything.) I answered, "Sure, why not?" It was winter, and he told me that he was concerned her inhalers might not work at high altitude or if they got very cold because of the low temperatures. "What do you think?" he asked me.

I wasn't sure if aerosols would function promptly. (Dry powdered inhalers are now available so this would no longer be an issue.) I suggested that his daughter tie a string around her inhaler and wear it around her neck under her clothes where it would remain warm. I was just patting myself on the back about this creative solution when I got the next phone call, an angry one from Erin's mother. It turned out her parents were divorced, her mother had custody, and she did not want her daughter to go mountain climbing with anyone, let alone her ex-husband. Sometimes allergy and asthma management has nothing to do with the patient!

Almost anything your child wants to do is possible. As you'll see in this chapter, certain activities require some pre-thinking and preparation, but if you've thought it through, almost anything from a sleepover to a wintertime trip up Mount Rainier ought to be possible.

Sleepovers

Sleepovers are rites of passage for children, and it's very important that a child with allergies or asthma participate in them just like his friends. Generally, they aren't too much of a problem, but every now and then the invitation may come from a child with three cats—and your child is highly allergic—or a family too disorganized to count on to give your child his medicine at the right time. (If they aren't willing to share this responsibility, there are probably other good reasons why your child shouldn't sleep there.)

Children pick up on parental attitudes about things, and if you communicate that you're nervous about your daughter sleeping at someone else's home, that concern will transfer to her. It's important to be open-minded about these experiences and demonstrate to your child how she can take care of herself when away from home. The key to a successful sleepover is to plan ahead. Talk to the other parents about any concerns you have. Pack medications in a clear sealable bag with a brief note outlining when and how to give each medication.

Some parents and children seem embarrassed about their medical conditions and try to keep them secret. This isn't a good idea. Kids need to learn to be matter-of-fact about these kinds of things. If they learn to take them in stride, their friends will, too. I often have patients who tell me that sometimes their friends will remind them to take their medications.

Key Point: *Always send medications with your child on sleepovers. An allergy or asthma attack away from home is frightening and embarrassing.*

Not every sleepover is possible. If you know your child is allergic to cats, for instance, be wary of homes with cats. As discussed in Chapter 9, cats spread their allergens all over carpeting, sofas, and beds. It doesn't do much good to keep the cat out of the bedroom for one night since cat allergens will remain for weeks. You may want to encourage the kids to sleep more frequently at your home.

Summer Camp

When I first started in practice, summer camp presented major problems. Asthma and allergies were not as frequently recognized, and camps were not set up to deal with these issues properly. Fortunately, this has changed. All well-established accredited summer camps have excellent nurses on staff and established policies and procedures to keep track of your child's medical issues and medications. Check the camp literature or inquire about the camp health policies before you sign your child up for a session, but I feel reasonably comfortable telling you that all camps take medical issues seriously.

Despite this, I fully understand how frightening that first summer camp experience is for both my patients and their parents. Planning and preparation are key. Set up an appointment with your physician in April or May, and develop a plan for summer camp. Discuss how an asthma attack or severe allergies should be handled. Many kids are bothered by allergies and asthma in the spring and fall and have relatively quiet periods during July and early August. Often medications can be decreased between those two seasons, but this may be a mistake for a child going away for camp, particularly for the first time. Sometimes it is safer to continue a preventive regimen all summer. Because most camps are in the woods, a common allergy problem is mold. Mold loves to grow in wet leaves, and mold spores blow all over camp. If your child is allergic to mold, make sure the camp counselors and managers have a clear plan if her allergies act up while there.

If you drive your child to camp, meet with the health office staff and give them the medicines yourself. If you can't personally deliver your child to camp, ask a camp representative how to be certain the nurse gets your child's medications and instructions.

Give your child's physician(s) permission to discuss your child's health with the camp nurses, and make sure the camp lets you know what is going on. In my experience, camp nurses are fabulous, love hearing from me, and are always very open to my suggestions.

Family Trips

I'm not sure why, but kids tend to get sick when they are traveling. One can't help but wonder about airplane air, though I have never seen any scientific studies about this issue. Perhaps stress or changes in routines and sleep patterns make the difference. It is far better to bring adequate medications and not need them than to be away from home unprepared.

Key Point: *Young kids frequently get sick while traveling, so always be prepared.*

The most common problems usually involve young children who are being treated with medications given in a nebulizer, a commonly used device explained in detail in the next chapter. Nebulizers are often bulky and heavy; many parents are tempted to leave them home if the child hasn't needed it in a few months. This is a mistake. If your child might possibly need a nebulizer, take it along. If you are traveling outside the United States, make sure your machine will work wherever you are going. Outlets are often designed differently in many countries, and both the current and voltage may be different. All of these factors need to be considered in advance. Some nebulizers work with batteries, and this type of machine is a great choice for frequent travelers. (Be sure you take along plenty of extra fresh batteries.) If your child's asthma can be controlled by using an inhaler, you won't need to travel with a nebulizer, but don't switch your child over for the first time while traveling.

If you need help, advice, or even medication while you are away, call your doctor. Fortunately, in the United States, physicians are permitted to call prescriptions into pharmacies in states other than where we are licensed. (When you call, have ready the telephone number of a pharmacy near where you are staying in case the doctor wants to call in a prescription.) While cell phones have greatly eased the issue of a doctor being able to return your call, you may be in a bad signal area or may not have your phone with you, so also leave your hotel phone number and specify the times when you will be there.

Mountain Climbing and Snow Sports in High Altitudes

The effects of high altitude on health are complex, and an in-depth discussion is not appropriate for this book. However, because of the popularity of mountain climbing and snow-related sports like skiing, I am frequently asked about the specific problems children with asthma may have at high altitude, so let me make a few comments.

Poorly controlled asthma will worsen symptoms associated with high altitude. The number one problem is that the amount of oxygen in the air at high altitudes is lower than at sea level. If the oxygen level in your blood is already low, you will have less reserve if it drops even further. Therefore, you are more likely to develop symptoms associated with low oxygen, such as headaches, fatigue, muscle aches, dizziness, or sleepiness. The second problem is that people with poorly controlled asthma are at greater risk of developing true high altitude or mountain sickness, which rarely occurs at less than 10,000 to 12,000 feet. This is a potentially life-threatening illness in anyone with or without asthma, but may be worse in someone with asthma. With high-altitude sickness, fluid builds up in your lungs, making you very short of breath. This is called *pulmonary edema*. If this occurs you must quickly seek medical attention, and almost certainly you will have to go back to a lower altitude as soon as possible.

If your child's asthma is well controlled then they probably are at no higher risk for these problems than anyone else. So if your child with asthma is going to a high altitude, be certain her asthma is under superb control and that she faithfully takes her asthma medications. Finally, with or without asthma, carefully follow all expert advice about proper acclimation procedures.

Scuba Diving

Scuba diving is a tough issue. Anyone who takes up this sport must understand that there is a small but real associated risk, with or without asthma. It is estimated that between fifty and one hundred people die each year in the United States while diving, and asthma may increase this risk. The number one concern is air suddenly leaking out of the lungs into the space between your lungs and your rib cage. This condition, called *pneumothorax*, results in partial lung collapse and is not uncommon with severe asthma attacks. Pneumothorax must be promptly treated and could be potentially disastrous if it occurs underwater.

For this reason, many groups and agencies that certify scuba divers will refuse to certify people with active asthma. Some will only certify with approval from a physician. Every pulmonologist sooner or later must deal with this issue, though many are reluctant, in part due to concern over the medico-legal issues—getting sued—if something goes wrong.

Since asthma is so common and mild cases go unrecognized, it is safe to say that many people with asthma have taken up scuba without difficulty. My approach is to explain the risks to people with asthma or their parents and emphasize that they are taking a risk and that no physician can change that. If you let your children ride a motorcycle, the same rules apply.

Many parents are not aware of the problems of scuba diving, so spread the word. Just recently I got a call from Mrs. Labrietta, whose fourteen-year-old son, Tony, had been a patient of mine with mild asthma for many years. He had not been back to see me for many years, as his parents thought he had outgrown his asthma. They were scheduled to go on a family trip in four days, and they had registered Tony for a five-day scuba certification course. To their surprise, their pediatrician felt uncomfortable signing the medical release form and suggested they bring Tony in to see me. Lo and behold, despite his denial of symptoms, pulmonary function tests confirmed that he really hadn't completely outgrown his asthma, and in fact it was not advisable for Tony to dive that week. The only responsible medical decision was to not sign the consent form. The best time to find out about one's physical preparedness for scuba diving is not a few days before an expensive prepaid trip to the Caribbean. There are differences of opinion, but most experts agree on the following:

- There is little point in restricting asthmatics to just shallow water diving, including snuba diving, a form of diving that is more advanced than snorkling but less complex than scuba diving. The pressure gradients are great enough in just a few feet of water to create the setting for pneumothorax.

- If your child's asthma is active, I don't think it is wise to let her dive. Active means any symptoms at all within a few weeks or months. My advice is to enjoy snorkeling.

- If your child has a history of asthma and has had no symptoms for at least a few years, an evaluation by a pediatric pulmonologist is in order, with performance of pulmonary function tests. Some experts also recommend X-rays of the chest. If there are any abnormalities in either pulmonary function tests or X-rays, it's probably not advisable to dive.

TAKE-HOME MESSAGES

- Sleepovers, summer camp, and family trips are all perfectly manageable. Doing a little research ahead of time will let you make adequate preparations for your child so that she can enjoy doing absolutely everything any other child would be permitted to do.

- Bring all of your child's medicines whenever he leaves home for an extended time, even if you don't expect to need them.

- Trips are not the best time to risk stopping daily medications.

- Mountain climbing and scuba diving entail increased risks. Discuss these issues with your child's asthma specialist—hopefully not the day before you are planning to leave.

PART FOUR:

ASTHMA ACTION PLAN: MEDICATION AND TREATMENT

THIRTEEN

ASTHMA:
OVERVIEW OF TREATMENT

Five-year-old Adam came to see me with his mother, father, maternal grandmother, and two older sisters. They piled into my office, and as usual I asked why they were here. Adam had been coughing for a long time, but they couldn't agree on how long. "When's the last time you remember him going a week without coughing?" I asked. Grandma and Dad couldn't remember. Mom thought that maybe he had a good week last summer, but she wasn't certain. I asked what their pediatrician had thought about the matter. They couldn't really tell me, but they had tried all kinds of stuff for his cough: antibiotics, prescription cough medicines, over-the-counter cough syrups, homeopathic remedies, chiropractic, and, one time out of desperation, Grandma had taken him to Florida in the hopes that hot weather would do the trick. But if anything ever helped, they couldn't really remember.

After my evaluation was complete, I knew that Adam had asthma. His primary care physicians had considered that diagnosis, but their first attempts at using asthma medications didn't work. And since he never wheezed, they had gone on to other approaches. His coughing waxed and waned for months and Adam's family felt frustrated and defeated. Coughing can be very tough to control, and most of the time there is no underlying serious illness, it's just the medicines haven't worked. I reassured Adam's family, told them we were going to stop this cough, and that together we would learn what it takes to control it in the future. I don't think they quite believed me, until Adam's cough disappeared within a few days of that first visit. What a relief!

In this chapter I am going to review how to design an effective treatment strategy for your child with asthma.

Asthma is a chronic condition, every child is different and there may be a lot of trial and error in finding the best approach. The plan will vary with age, your child's particular asthma triggers, and perhaps each season. Also remember that as our understanding of asthma expands, medicines improve and treatment philosophy evolves. So discuss with your doctor not a lifelong plan but one that makes sense for your child for a reasonable period of time, such as for the next one or two seasons. That's one of the reasons I always insist on follow-up visits at least every six months.

Key Point: *Kids change, so their medications must change along with them.*

DETERMINING YOUR CHILD'S ASTHMA PLAN

STEP #1: Clarify goals for your child's asthma.

STEP #2: Decide on daily "preventive" medication or just "as needed" medication.

STEP #3: Choose oral or inhaled medications.

STEP #4: Decide which method of inhalation would be best.

STEP #5: Choose a controller or maintenance regimen.

STEP #6: Choose "reliever" medications.

STEP #7: Consider additional medications if intermittent short-acting beta-adrenergic agents are inadequate.

STEP #8: Clarify how and when to start, increase, or decrease medications.

STEP #9: Don't leave the office without a plan for emergencies.

STEP #10: Plan follow-up visits.

STEP #1:
Clarify goals for your child's asthma.

Key Point: *The most important step is to figure out your goals.*

When we think about health issues, most families—and many physicians—don't think about setting goals, yet it's as important in medicine as it is at school or in business. You can only assess your success if you have clear goals. The most important thing I do is help parents talk out what they actually want from medications and encourage them to analyze at each visit whether the plan is meeting their needs, and if not, why not.

Just this past week I met with a mother and son for a six-month checkup. When I asked how he was doing, Mom answered, "Not very well." Naturally I felt like a failure and wanted to know what happened. "Did he have a lot of wheezing?" I asked. "No," she said. "Did he have a lot of coughing?" "No, not really." "Miss a lot of school?" Proudly she told me he had no absences all year. Baffled, I asked her why she thought he wasn't doing well. She told me that he has a chronic runny or stuffy nose, walks around with a fistful of tissues, and is constantly clearing his throat. I looked at my last notes, and all I had prescribed was an asthma inhaler. So I asked her what she'd been doing for his nasal symptoms. And she said, "Nothing." Clearly at the last visit, she and I had not communicated properly about goals.

Let me repeat some of the important goals I have previously suggested:

Goal #1:   I don't want asthma to affect a child's lifestyle.

Goal #2:   Any cough or chest congestion that your child develops from an upper-respiratory-tract infection should be completely gone within about two weeks.

One key to success in managing asthma is to get a patient back to "perfect" after an illness. And when I say perfect, I mean perfect; not just that a doctor says that your child's chest is clear. I mean that your son or daughter should have no cough, no rattle, no shortness of breath when running around . . . perfect; as good as they are in the middle of July. This often does not happen. Millions of children walk around with a mild, low-level cough and chest congestion in between colds, especially during the school year. They aren't really sick but they aren't perfect either. This is bad and I'm going to tell you why.

When a child's bronchial tubes are 10 to 20 percent narrowed, they may have no obvious wheezing and will be able to participate in all activities, but they will have less reserve. The next trigger that comes along might bring the tubes to a 30 to 40 percent narrowing, and suddenly they are likely to have significant symptoms. If, however, their lung function before they are exposed to a trigger is perfect—100 percent—then if the tubes narrow 20 percent they will only have mild symptoms, such as cough, congestion, or mild chest tightness, and you'll be very pleased that their asthma is mild.

Key Point: *By changing the baseline, your child's asthma will be milder.*

The second reason it's so important to get back to perfect in between illnesses is that while your child may seem "pretty well," they really could feel a lot better. There may be vague complaints: excess mucus may be swallowed, and this leads to reflux (heartburn), chest pains, stomachaches, gas, constipation, or irregularity. In addition, chronic, low-level, partially treated bronchospasm has subtle but undeniable side effects. Children may not sleep as well; they may not wake up feeling as rested; they may not dream as much; they may not be as alert in school; their attention span may be less than it should be. They may not be able to run quite as fast, may be more winded with simple activities. On a scale from one to ten, they're just not a ten.

Finally, it is well documented that chronic inflammation and low-level bronchospasm may permanently scar lungs; when you study people who have had asthma for more than ten or twenty years, they no longer have normal function. Their bronchial tubes are now permanently narrowed, or to use the popular expression in the medical literature, "remodeled." Unfortunately, since our airways are constantly exposed to the outside world, we all develop a mild degree of permanent narrowing and scarring as we age. Our job as parents and physicians, I believe, is to get our children through their childhood with the best possible lung function, so that we can send them into adult life as a perfect ten.

Goal #3: No side effects from medications. None.
Goal #4: Use the least amount of medications to achieve goals #1, 2, and 3.

No matter how safe a medication is, there is no such thing as a medication that works that doesn't also have at least some small risk. No parent wants to give their child medications, but treating asthma is very important to your child's life. We should continuously reevaluate and ask if we can't do just as well with less. That's another reason I insist on routine visits, usually at least every six months.

SUGGESTED GOALS FOR ASTHMA THERAPY

Goal #1: I don't want asthma to affect a child's lifestyle.
Goal #2: Any cough or chest congestion from an upper-respiratory-tract infection should be completely gone within about two weeks.
Goal #3: No side effects from medications. None.
Goal #4: Use the least amount of medications to achieve goals #1, 2, and 3.

How I Explain Asthma to a Child

My explanation varies with the developmental stage of the child, but in general, I try to convey that what is happening is not mysterious or scary—it can be described, treated, and controlled. If I were talking to a pre-adolescent, my explanation would be something along the following lines:

There is absolutely nothing wrong with your lungs. They are working great and will last at least 150 years! Asthma is not a problem with your actual lungs but with the bronchial tubes that bring the air in and out. These bronchial tubes have branches just like an upside down tree:

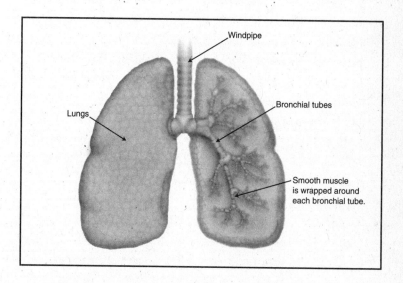

Windpipe

Bronchial tubes

Lungs

Smooth muscle is wrapped around each bronchial tube.

All of us have muscle built into the walls of the bronchial tubes, just like muscles everywhere else in your body. This muscle is there to protect our lungs from all of the stuff that floats around in the air: pollution, cigarette smoke, germs, pollen, everything. Whenever we breathe something in that doesn't belong in our lungs, three things happen: (1) We cough trying to get out whatever landed on the walls of the tubes. (2) We produce mucus that surrounds any particles that we have breathed in, making it easier to cough them out. (3) The muscles in the walls of the bronchial tubes constrict and the tubes narrow, trying to protect themselves. When your bronchial tubes constrict or narrow a little bit, you may feel "tight" in the chest. When they narrow a lot you may feel short of breath and hear a wheezing sound. Cough, mucus, spasm; all humans have these important defenses.

Actually everyone coughs a little bit every day! *Asthma* simply means that your bronchial tubes are just a little more sensitive than mine. If anyone breathes in enough cigarette smoke, for instance, they will cough, produce mucus, and wheeze. But people with asthma will react to just a little bit of smoke, while other people won't cough or wheeze until a lot of smoke is inhaled. If I put enough dog hair down anyone's bronchial tubes, they will react. Some people cough with just one hair, some won't cough or feel "tight" unless they breathe in at least ten hairs, and other people won't cough unless you put the whole dog down there. Just like some people are tall and some people are short, some people have bronchial tubes or airways that are more sensitive or hyperreactive.

In my opinion, asthma is not a disease. It is merely a condition in which your bronchial tubes or airways are just a little more sensitive than they should be. Lots of people have mild asthma and don't even know it—you're lucky because we know what you have and now we can treat it so that you can do anything you want to do.

STEP #2:
Decide on daily "preventive" medication or just "as needed" medication.

While many children with asthma can be adequately managed with medication just when needed, many cannot. Ironically, you may avoid the strongest medications by keeping your child on much lower doses on a daily basis, and only increasing medications for occasional exacerbations. It's important to make a rational decision based on your own child's asthma and their triggers. Sometimes it's easy. If the only time your child ever has asthma symptoms is when she is participating in sports that really get her heart and lungs pumping, she may not need daily medicine. Using some type of inhaler fifteen minutes before sports or gym class should prevent her from having exercise-induced symptoms. In this case, the goal for treatment (ability to participate in sports) has been met with a very small (least amount) of medication.

Your teenage daughter may only have coughing, chest congestion, or wheezing with colds, and at this point in her life, she only really gets one or two colds each school year. In that case you may be able to achieve your goals just by starting medications as soon as she starts to cough. She can be kept on the medications for the week to ten days it might take for the viral infection to run its course. Therefore, this asthmatic condition may be kept under control with medicine given only as needed. However, medicine given just as needed won't work well in a younger child who is likely to suffer six or eight or more respiratory infections from September to June. If each one lasts more than a week, clearly this child would be better off on a preventive daily regimen, since as needed medication might be needed almost every day anyway.

If allergies play an important role in your child's asthma, then during the seasons when her allergies are triggered her asthma will be triggered every day, and preventive medicines make the most sense. If a child suffers serious asthma attacks, gets sick enough to require hospitalization, emergency room visits, or frequent courses of such strong medicines as oral corticosteroids (prednisone), then daily preventive medication may be safest. It is important to remember that, though rare, asthma can kill. Prevention of severe attacks is extremely important!

Parents know that infants and young children can go from really well to really sick really fast. Because they have smaller bronchial tubes and immature immune systems, they may run into difficulties before medications have time to take effect (many of these medications take at least a few days to be effective). For this reason, the as-needed approach just may not be adequate for some young children—be sure to keep reevaluating as you may be able to switch later on.

Now you are ready to choose specific medications. Remember, these decisions are not engraved in stone. If your first approach doesn't work, change it.

PREVENTIVE VS. AS-NEEDED THERAPY

Preventive therapy

Advantages	Disadvantages	When to Consider
Works better	Requires daily medication even when well	When triggers are frequent or attacks are severe

As-needed therapy

Advantages	Disadvantages	When to Consider
Allows your child to be off medication in between episodes	Your child will have more symptoms when they are triggered	When there are long breaks between episodes

STEP #3:
Choose oral or inhaled medications.

This used to be a simple question. Over the last fifteen years inhaled medications have been preferred because they deliver medication directly to the lungs without any delay in onset and without the side effects that used to occur with older oral medications. Remember, anything that is swallowed has to be absorbed into the bloodstream and then must travel through the body to have an effect. Therefore, as a general rule, inhaled medications are safer and faster-acting than oral medications.

There are, however, exceptions. Inhaled steroids, which we will discuss at length in this chapter, may cause side effects at high doses despite the fact that they are inhaled. And some of the newer oral asthma medicines such as Accolate and Singulair, known as leukotriene modifiers, really are extraordinarily safe. So while it is still true that inhaled medications are faster-acting, not all oral medications have significant side effects.

STEP #4:
Decide which method of inhalation would be best.

If you and your physicians choose inhaled medications, just as important as choosing a specific drug is choosing how that drug is delivered. There are four basic ways to deliver inhaled medications:

Nebulizers

What most people refer to as a "nebulizer" is really made up of two parts: an air compressor that generates a flow of air through a tube into a specially designed plastic "nebulizer cup," which actually breaks the liquid into a fine mist of particles small enough to be inhaled into the lungs. The speed of nebulization depends on both the strength of the compressor and the design of the nebulizer cup. Most standard nebulizers take between eight and fifteen minutes to complete one treatment. They also aren't very convenient. Plug-in models are most common, but portable ones with battery packs and ones that plug into the car cigarette lighter are also available. In addition, many preventive or controller medications are not available for nebulization, so this method severely limits a family's choices. Many nebulizers are pretty noisy. Faster, smaller, quieter nebulizers are available, but they are expensive and may break down more easily. If you want to use a nebulizer but your child has difficulty sitting still for the time required to nebulize medications, ask your physicians to help you obtain a faster and quieter machine. Health insurance companies don't always understand, but the difference between a fast, quiet, and expensive nebulizer and a slow, noisy, inexpensive machine may be the difference between success and failure. If your physician is recommending a nebulizer, ask about the pros and cons of different machines. This offers your medical professional the opportunity to consider exactly what would be best for your child. For instance, if a child is going to require medication in more than one place or even in the car on the go, a portable nebulizer may be a good approach. If you don't need portability, a nebulizer that simply plugs into the wall will work well. Then, as I mentioned in Chapter 12, there is the issue of traveling outside the United States. Without an adapter, the differences in voltage and electric cycles can really do a number on a nebulizer.

I am reminded of Jill, a bright Ivy League college student who called me from her hotel in Vienna. Jill told me that she smelled burning and there was smoke coming from her compressor, and what did I think she should do? The first thing I asked was whether she had unplugged her machine. "No, should I?" she asked. So I said, "Jill, put down the phone and go unplug the machine before you burn down the hotel."

Our conversation turned to the question of where she could get a new nebulizer in Vienna. I suggested she check the closest pharmacy. As it happens, she found a wonderful, small, fast, and quiet nebulizer. I was so impressed by it that for years I recommended that brand to my patients.

The vast majority of children today do not require a nebulizer. However, it can be very useful for certain children who just need occasional reliever medications (discussed later in the chapter) rather than daily controller medications.

HOW TO USE A NEBULIZER

1. Make sure the nebulizer cup is clean and in good condition.
2. Connect one end of the long tubing to the nebulizer cup and the other end to the air compressor. Make sure the connections are tight.
3. Fill the cup with the appropriate medications. Be careful not to spill any.
4. Plug in the compressor (if needed) and turn it on.
5. Have your child breathe normally while receiving a treatment. There is no reason for any special breathing technique.
6. Older kids may be able to properly use a mouthpiece. If so, more medicine will get into the lungs.
7. Younger children will have to use a mask. Make sure the mask is sized properly to comfortably fit over your child's nose and mouth.

8. If your child won't sit still for a mask, you will have no choice but to just aim the plume of smoke at their face. Good luck!
9. When you are done, follow the directions for proper cleaning. Most models are dishwasher safe.

METERED DOSE INHALERS

Metered dose inhalers (MDI) release a specific amount of medication each time you spray. The device consists of a mouthpiece and a canister of pressurized medication that fits into a plastic sleeve. They are a handy but ineffective product, and I do not prescribe them without some sort of spacer device. When you spray most available inhalers, the mist moves at roughly sixty-five miles per hour, and very little of it will turn the corner in your mouth and get down into the bronchial tubes, leaving most of the medication coating the tongue and back of the throat and doing little to open your child's airways.

I know you see lots of people carrying their little inhalers and puffing them directly into their mouths. Many physicians, particularly physicians for adults, have not really gotten this message. Many of my patients seem to think that once their child gets old enough, they can start using their inhaler directly into their mouth. In my opinion you are never old enough for this method to be recommended.

Key Point: **Inhalers sprayed into the mouth are very inefficient. Always use a spacer.**

METERED DOSE INHALERS WITH A
SPACER DEVICE OR HOLDING CHAMBER

Spacers or holding chambers are the key to success with inhalers. While the difference between these two devices is explained below, the basic concept is that the medicine is held in such a way that the person using it can inhale the medicine more slowly, rather than having it speed into the mouth so quickly it never makes it down into the lungs. The development of these devices is what made inhalers so successful. Most holding chambers have a mouthpiece, but in my experience children under the age of five or six often are not able to maintain a tight seal with the mouthpiece and inhale adequately. A major advance in pediatric asthma care is the development of holding chambers with a mask instead of a mouthpiece. This invention allows metered dose inhalers to be used in children of all ages and neurological development, including the tiniest premature infant.

There is a subtle difference between a spacer and a holding chamber. A spacer is an attachment shaped like the cardboard in a toilet paper roll that attaches to an inhaler and keeps it a couple of inches away from your mouth. While this helps aim the spray better, it is not as good as a holding chamber, of which there are now many brands. A holding chamber attaches to all inhalers and holds the mist for a few seconds, allowing the patient to inhale the mist at a slower flow rate and thereby assure more effective delivery of medication into the lungs. Unfortunately, many health insurance plans do not pay for these gizmos, which I consider essential. What amazes me even more is the wide range of prices charged for holding chambers in retail pharmacies. In the New York area, for instance, most patients are charged $30–$40 for an Aerochamber, and some of my patients have complained to me of paying

$65 or $75. I now know of one web site at which you can buy the same device for $18! It's worth shopping around.

Many companies are now making holding chambers, but there are remarkably few studies comparing different brands. The only studies I'm aware of suggested that the bigger the chamber the better. However, what the chamber is made of may be more important. If there is a tiny electrostatic charge at the inner surface of the device, medicine may cling to the walls, allowing less to be inhaled. One model of holding chamber, Vortex, takes this into account and is now available in the United States. These details are minor compared to the tremendous benefit of using any sort of spacer device.

Metered dose inhalers have a major drawback: They rely on a chemical propellant and most of them still use CFCs (chlorofluorocarbons), which are bad for the ozone layer. For too long, inhaled asthma medications have been exempt from international treaties designed to get rid of these chemicals, but now the American pharmaceutical industry is required to faze them out. Not only are they bad for the environment, but I'm not crazy about asking all of my patients to inhale that stuff into their lungs. I, for one, feel mildly tremulous after I inhale that stuff, a side effect I suspect many patients attribute erroneously to the actual medication, not the propellant.

Chlorofluorocarbon propellants are now being replaced with a newer safer type, called HFAs (hydrofluoroalkanes). These newer inhalers require less propellant, result in a slower flow rate, and are safe for the environment. Their valves don't clog easily and it isn't necessary to shake these inhalers. If an older child has mastered an unhurried technique with one of these newer inhalers, then a reasonable amount of medicine will be inhaled without a spacer, though I still prefer a holding chamber.

HOW TO USE AN MDI WITH
A HOLDING CHAMBER

1. Make sure the inhaler isn't empty.
2. Make sure the holding chamber is in good condition, with no leaks.
3. Insert inhaler firmly into chamber.
4. Activate the inhaler, discharging one spray into the chamber.
5. The preferred technique is to coach your child to inhale as slowly and completely as possible, followed by at least a five second breath-hold. Some models whistle if your child is breathing too quickly.
6. For young children who are not able to master this technique, simply encourage your child to complete at least five normal, quiet, easy breaths after each spray.
7. Repeat this procedure for each spray as directed by your child's physician.

DRY POWDER INHALERS

The newest inhalers sweeping the asthma market deliver medication as a dry powder. These inhalers have no propellant. The patient seals her lips around the mouthpiece and withdraws the medication herself. This is a very efficient and elegant design that improves the delivery of medication without a bulky holding chamber. Not all patients and their physicians understand that the inhalation technique is different from that with a metered dose inhaler and holding chamber. The optimal technique with a holding chamber is to inhale very slowly, allowing as much medicine as possible to be delivered deep into your lungs. With a dry powdered inhaler, you need to inhale quickly. Actually, most people rush their inhalation anyway, so this is an advantage for dry powder inhalers.

Another advantage to dry powder inhalers is that it is easier to tell when they are empty. This sounds trivial, but it's actually quite helpful. It is more difficult to discern whether a standard inhaler is full or empty, and sometimes a child's asthma veers out of control because they've been puffing on an empty inhaler.

I am still skittish about recommending these inhalers to children younger than seven to nine years of age. Despite their best efforts to hold the mouthpiece properly and inhale with enough force to get their full dose, most young children are not ready to master this technique. MDIs with a holding chamber remain my first choice for young children.

If your child is truly allergic to milk, you have to be wary of dry powder inhalers because they all contain lactose. Lactose is a sugar that does not trigger allergic reactions. However, lactose is derived from milk and no manufacturer can guarantee that tiny amounts of milk protein haven't slipped through the process that extracts lactose from milk.

FREQUENCY OF ROUTINE INHALED MEDICATION

When your doctor is working out a medical regimen for your child, be sure to consider the complexity of the plan. If it is very complicated, requiring medications to be taken three or four times per day, that may not be practical. How will you accomplish that? When will that middle dose be given at school and by whom? Will your child have to go to the nurse every day? Consider how this may affect a child's ability to participate in activities—and remember that anything that singles out a child for separate treatment is socially ostracizing. No child wants to be sitting in the nurse's office waiting for medication. If one goal is that your child's asthma shouldn't affect her lifestyle, then a complex routine is already one strike against success.

The practicalities of a regimen may be problematic if your child divides his time between two homes. It is very important that divorced parents agree on the plan.

STEP #5:
Choose a controller or maintenance regimen.

For children receiving daily preventive therapy, a controller regimen needs to be established. (If your child is taking medication only as needed, skip to the next step.) There are now a variety of medications designed to be given preventively, with new ones arriving daily. In fact, by the time this book is published, there probably will be a couple of new ones on the market that I haven't yet heard of. So by and large I am going to try to emphasize categories of medications. There are slight advantages and disadvantages among competing brands within these categories, but these differences are much less important than the distinctions among the categories.

Important Reminder

"Controllers" are medications given every day, regardless of how your child feels. They are not given for immediate relief of symptoms. For immediate relief, use a "reliever."

INHALED STEROIDS

Inhaled steroids are generally the best type of daily therapy for the majority of children with asthma. These are excellent anti-inflammatory agents, and their development has revolutionized our treatment of asthma. Known as glucocorticosteroids, these drugs are not at all like the steroids athletes sometimes abuse, and they do not have the same list of side effects. All of

the glucocorticosteroids are copies of cortisol, a naturally occurring hormone we all have in our bloodstream. When used
in appropriate doses, inhaled steroids are really very safe and
are by far the most effective first line for chronic preventive
therapy. By appropriate doses, I mean the lowest dose possible
to meet your goals. At low doses, the risks are really very
small, and remember that the risks of chronic inadequately
treated asthma are much, much greater.

The side effect parents and pediatricians are most concerned about is growth failure, which is an unequivocal side
effect of long-term use of oral steroids such as prednisone.
Since inhaling steroids allows us to use much smaller doses,
it was hoped that we would not see this effect with the inhaled route. And in fact, at the most common doses used, we
really do not see this problem. Some children have such severe asthma that they require doses that are two, three, and
four times the average, and growth can be slowed at these
high doses. This isn't as simple to figure out as you might
think, as severe asthma itself slows growth! In addition, many
of these same children often require multiple and prolonged
courses of oral steroids. While at high doses we know that inhaled steroids can slow growth in some children, as of this
writing, the preponderance of data suggests that even with
high doses eventual final adult height is really not changed.
Inhaled steroids are dramatically safer than oral steroids.

Key Point: *Low doses of inhaled steroids*
are very safe and effective. It
is important to try to lower the
dose when possible.

The choice of inhaled steroid is mostly dependent on
which inhalation technique seems best for your child. For in-

stance, if you choose nebulization, only one brand is available in the United States. Dry powder inhalers only come in two brands. However, there are many brands of metered dose inhalers available.

The list of medications in this category keeps expanding. Most specialists agree that differences between brands are less impressive in reality than as they are portrayed, and scientists have even had difficulty agreeing on their relative potency. Following is the current list of medications in this category.

Key Point: *In each table that follows, I have listed all brand names available in the United States as of this writing. Many are manufactured in several formulations (solutions, syrups, tablets, inhalers, etc.) and some of the older brands are being phased out, so check with your doctor or pharmacist to see what is currently available.*

CURRENTLY AVAILABLE INHALED
CORTICOSTEROIDS

Generic Names	Brand Names
beclomethasone	Qvar
budesonide	Pulmicort
flunisolide	Aerobid
fluticasone	Flovent and Advair, which is Flovent combined with Serevent
triamcinolone	Azmacort

CHROMONES

Chromones appear to be the safest of all controller medications. They are derived from plants and have essentially no significant side effects. Two drugs are currently available and one of them, cromolyn sodium, is the more popular of the two in the United States. Available in generic form, this medication is known by the brand name Intal. Doctors are as prone to fashion as anyone, and cromolyn is out of style. However, in the right situation it can be an excellent alternative.

Cromolyn is available as both a nebulizer solution and as a metered dose inhaler, so any child can use it. The bad news is that at currently accepted doses, cromolyn just isn't that great and is not as effective as even low doses of inhaled steroids. In addition, it takes at least three or four weeks of daily inhalation of cromolyn before the preventive effect is optimized, so you really have to be organized and start your child on this medication well in advance of when it is needed. For instance, when I used to prescribe a lot of cromolyn, I would instruct parents to begin giving it to their children two or three weeks *before* school started each fall. This is not necessary with inhaled steroids.

I believe that the number one reason cromolyn failed to prevent asthma attacks is that kids were not taking it properly. In my experience, cromolyn doesn't work well unless a child inhales it at least three or—better yet—four times each day. I suspect that children doing well on twice daily cromolyn may not need a control medication at all.

If used properly, with parents highly motivated to use the safest medication possible, preventive therapy with cromolyn can work. Sometimes, though, even when used properly, cromolyn just isn't up to the task.

The second drug in the chromone family is nedocromil, available in either generic form or by its brand name, Tilade. This is an excellent European medication that never took off in the United States, mostly because of inadequate market-ing. Nedocromil used with a holding chamber can effectively control mild asthma, to some degree, without significant side effects, but it is not currently available in the United States.

CURRENTLY AVAILABLE CHROMONES

Generic Names	Brand Names
cromolyn sodium	Intal
nedocromil	Tilade

LEUKOTRIENE MODIFIERS

There are now three drugs on the market in this category, Zyflo, Accolate, and Singulair. Accolate and Singulair are very popular, and as a result we have developed a lot of experience with these two medications in a relatively short time. Zyflo has not taken off and I have no experience with it.

Similar to chromones and corticosteroids, these medications also inhibit the inflammatory process in the airways, but by a different mechanism. While corticosteroids treat a variety of inflammatory diseases including rheumatoid arthritis and kidney disease, leukotriene modifiers have a more focused approach and work to reduce only the inflammation associated with allergic reactions. Because of these limited effects, these medications appear to be safer than inhaled steroids. Unfortunately they are often not as effective. (There is no such thing as a free lunch.)

Singulair is taken as either a chewable or regular tablet, and it is an exception to the rule that inhaled medications are safer than oral medications. The reason for its widespread use with children largely relies on the fact that both parents and physicians are delighted to have an alternative to inhaled steroids.

Although we now have good evidence that low doses of inhaled steroids are safe, many people continue to be afraid.

We are still learning a lot about these medications. One interesting characteristic of leukotriene modifiers is that some kids seem to respond well and others really don't. Research is being done to sort out why some patients are so-called responders and others are not. Generally speaking, if allergies are playing either a direct or indirect role in your child's symptoms, Singulair may help to some degree.

Accolate is another medication in this class, and some patients derive better asthma control with Accolate than Singulair. That's both the challenge and reward of caring for people—everyone is different.

Most patients with persistent asthma who require daily preventive therapy cannot be controlled with Singulair or Accolate alone. However, adding one of these medications to the regimen, as a so-called steroid-sparing agent, allows many children to achieve successful control with lower doses of steroids than otherwise possible.

Singulair and Accolate are now approved for treatment of the nasal symptoms of allergic rhinitis, though they may not be adequate by themselves. Since so many children with asthma also have chronic nasal congestion, this can be important.

CURRENTLY AVAILABLE
LEUKOTRIENE MODIFIERS

Generic Names	Brand Names
montelukast	Singulair
zafirlukast	Accolate
zileuton	Zyflo

LONG-ACTING INHALED
BETA-ADRENERGIC AGONISTS

Serevent and Foradil are relatively new to the American market but have been available elsewhere for some time. Unlike inhaled steroids, chromones, and leukotriene modifiers, these medications are not anti-inflammatory, and most experts agree they rarely should be used alone as daily controller medication. You may have heard about studies showing that when given alone these medications may make things worse. This is controversial, but what is not controversial is how many people have been able to get better control with lower steroid doses by adding these medications. Like the leukotriene modifiers, these medications are proving to be great additions to inhaled steroids, allowing kids to achieve their goals with lower steroid doses than would otherwise be possible. Although these drugs are chemically related to short-acting beta-adrenergic agonists, such as albuterol, that give fast relief, they are not appropriate for immediate relief. Serevent and Foradil are now only available as dry powder inhalers, so they cannot be used for young children or patients who cannot inhale deeply enough to properly actuate these devices. This is very frustrating since with their long duration of action these medications can be very helpful.

If low doses of inhaled steroids are not controlling your child's asthma, should you add a leukotriene modifier, such as Singulair or Accolate, or a long-acting beta agonist, such as Serevent or Foradil? As of this writing, this remains a very hot topic, with research studies on both sides of that debate. Suffice it to say that every child is different and you have to work with your doctor to identify which medicine works best.

CURRENTLY AVAILABLE LONG-ACTING
BETA-ADRENERGIC AGONISTS

<u>Generic Names</u>	<u>Brand Names</u>
formoterol	Foradil
salmeterol	Serevent and Advair, which is Serevent combined with Flovent

THEOPHYLLINE

Theophylline is taken orally, either as a capsule, syrup, or time-release "sprinkle" preparation. Before the avalanche of inhaled medications, theophylline was the mainstay of chronic preventive asthma care in the United States. Many of you may remember such products as SloPhyllin, Slobid, Theolair, and Theodur, and almost countless others, including newer ones such as Theo-24 and Uniphyl. So what happened? Well, when used alone, doses had to be pushed up so high that side effects became a real problem. In fact, at the levels required to control asthma when given alone, safety dictated following blood levels fairly closely, which was a hassle for everyone involved. In addition, with these high doses of theophylline, drug interactions needed to be watched carefully. A theophylline dose well tolerated under normal circumstances could become toxic when given with other medications.

I have decidedly mixed feelings about theophylline falling out of favor. On the one hand, inhaled steroids really are better overall. On the other hand, physicians today seem to have lost the use of some very good medications, and I believe that for some patients, theophylline still plays an important role. We no longer use theophylline as primary therapy for asthma, but rather as "add-on" therapy or a "steroid-sparing" agent. By adding theophylline to your child's regimen, asthma control can often be maintained with lower doses of inhaled steroids. And the beautiful thing about this approach is this allows us to use very low doses of theophylline. Low doses almost never cause side effects and blood levels aren't usually necessary.

CURRENTLY AVAILABLE BRANDS OF THEOPHYLLINE

Aerolate

Lufyllin

Theo-Dur

Uni-Dur

Uniphyl

FUTURE DIRECTIONS IN CONTROLLER MEDICATIONS

In the near future, I expect to see new controller medications. Like all of the medications discussed above, it will take some time before we know where they best fit into the management of children with asthma. Some of the new medications on the horizon are variations of the themes above and some are quite different, based on our increasingly sophisticated understanding of the inflammatory cascade of chemicals involved in allergies and asthma.

One of the most fascinating new approaches is the recently approved high-tech preventive medication called Xolair. This is a preventive therapy, given by injection every two to four weeks. This medication binds up any IgE floating around in the blood stream, blocking it from triggering an allergic cascade. (As you remember from Chapter 2, IgE is that all-important little molecule that is produced whenever someone is exposed to one of their specific allergens. This little antibody then triggers all of the symptoms of allergies.) This seems like a very exciting idea, and I hope it will allow us to prevent a lot of allergies and asthma altogether, avoiding the need for so many current medications. However, it is really too early to know if Xolair's potential will be realized. A second version of anti-IgE therapy is also being studied and hopefully will prove useful in the next few years.

CONTROLLER MEDICATIONS FOR ASTHMA

Category	Advantages	Disadvantages
Inhaled Steroids	Very effective Current best choice for most patients Anti-inflammatory	Significant long-term side effects at high doses
Chromones	Very safe, with long experience Mildly anti-inflammatory	Often inadequate Often requires frequent dosing
Long-acting Inhaled Beta-Adrenergic Agonists	Control symptoms of asthma very effectively Appear to be quite safe, but relatively new	Do not control the underlying inflammation, so probably should not be used alone Variable effectiveness, not everyone "responds"
Leukotriene Modifiers	Easy and convenient Effective against inflammation due to allergies	Often inadequate alone

Category	Advantages	Disadvantages
Theophylline	No significant long-term side effects	Significant immediate side effects at high doses
	Easy and convenient	Out of style
	Limited anti-inflammatory effects	
Anti-IgE Therapy	Could potentially prevent any significant allergic reaction, including asthma	Requires regular shots every two to four weeks
	First really new approach in many years	Won't help asthmatics who don't have allergies
		Expensive
		Long-term safety needs to be established

STEP #6:
Choose reliever medications.

For children who only need occasional asthma medication, the controller medications listed thus far are unnecessary. For immediate relief, choose something that works quickly and has no side effects. For the vast majority of children, this means choosing from a family of medications known as short-acting beta-adrenergic agents.

SHORT-ACTING BETA-ADRENERGIC AGONISTS

These medications are bronchodilators. That is, they directly relax the muscle spasm and therefore relieve the narrowing of the bronchial tubes that occur with asthma. There are a number of medications in this family, but albuterol is currently the most commonly used, and it is a good first choice for most children. (Those of us around more than twenty years ago do remember that there were other choices before albuterol was released, first as brand names, Ventolin and Proventil, and now in generic formulations.) Albuterol comes as a metered dose inhaler, nebulizer solution, syrup, and both short-acting and time-release tablets; each have their place. In general, the inhaled versions are preferred because there are fewer side effects at effective doses.

Many parents are convinced the metered dose inhaler is less effective than the nebulizer solution for at least two reasons: First, remember that without a holding chamber, metered dose inhalers don't deliver medication to the lungs very well. Second, we doctors have been at fault. For some strange reason, we continue to cling to the originally approved dose of two puffs of albuterol. In fact, if you take four to six puffs or even more, an albuterol inhaler in a holding chamber is just as good as a nebulizer, and maybe better. Sometimes I think the eleventh commandment passed down from Moses on Mount Sinai is that thou shalt use only two puffs of an inhaler. I wish this misunderstanding would fade by the time this book is published (but I doubt it).

Incidentally, albuterol was one of the first asthma medications to be released in the United States as a dry powder inhaler, Ventolin Rotacaps. I liked this formulation and so did my patients. Unfortunately, it is no longer available in America.

Proventil HFA is an albuterol inhaler that, unlike generic inhalers, is free of the CFC propellant that is bad for the environment.

Some children become jittery or sleepless, or they feel their heart beating quickly after inhaling albuterol. While side effects are rarely serious, they should not be tolerated. That is when your child should try other members of the short-acting beta-adrenergic family. Remember, there is no reason to put up with side effects.

I would be remiss if I didn't mention Primatine, which is the very popular over-the-counter inhaler that contains pure epinephrine. Epinephrine is a very effective bronchodilator, but it has major limitations. It works very quickly and wears off very quickly, which is why you see so many people puffing all day. And epinephrine has potentially far more side effects than any of the prescription bronchodilators, all of which were designed to improve upon epinephrine. With epinephrine, a prescription inhaler should be used.

There are newer additions to this family of fast-relief medications that I want to tell you about. The first is Maxair, which is pirbuterol, a drug very similar to albuterol. This medication is available in a cleverly designed inhaler called an Autohaler. This device is breath-activated, so a holding chamber is not necessary. Maxair Autohaler is a great option for portability if your kids are old enough to use it properly.

Xopenex is another important addition to the family of fast-acting relief medications. This medication is a purified cousin of albuterol, known as levalbuterol, which in most kids causes fewer side effects than albuterol. Whether it is any better or worse than plain old albuterol remains to be seen, but it is a great option for children who can't tolerate albuterol. Currently it is only available as a nebulizer solution.

CURRENTLY AVAILABLE SHORT-ACTING
BETA-ADRENERGIC AGENTS

Generic Names	Brand Names
albuterol	AccuNeb
	Combivent (combined with ipratroprium bromide)
	DuoNeb (combined with ipratroprium bromide)
	Proventil
	Ventolin
	Volmax
	VoSpire ER
isoetharine	Bronkosol
levalbuterol	Xopenex
metaproterenol	Alupent
pirbuterol	Maxair
terbutaline	Brethine

ANTICHOLINERGIC AGENTS

Ipratropium bromide (Atrovent) is a short-acting bronchodilator that works by a different mechanism, and its role in asthma care is still developing. This medication is available both as an MDI (alone and combined with albuterol, named Combivent) and in nebulizer vials (alone and mixed with albuterol, named DuoNeb), and it has traditionally been used by adults with chronic bronchitis.

Key Point: ***Atrovent and Combivent inhalers
both currently contain soy lecithin,
which is chemically related to soy
and peanuts. Therefore, children
who are known to have had severe
reactions to soy or peanuts are
cautioned not to use these inhalers.***

STEP #7:
Consider additional medications if intermittent short-acting beta-adrenergic agents are inadequate.

For many children, failure to control symptoms with as needed medication such as albuterol means that a continuous preventive approach should be considered. However, sometimes adding one or more of the controller medications for brief periods of time can help, avoiding the need for chronic preventive therapy.

In my practice we sometimes add inhaled steroids just for the duration of a viral respiratory tract infection (one or two weeks). This doesn't always work, especially with young children who get sick so quickly. Since this approach has not been adequately studied, it is not part of international treatment guidelines. But adding an inhaled steroid to a bronchodilator can sometimes help decrease coughing and excess mucus production.

Here's one more example: As will be discussed in chapter 16, a short-acting beta-adrenergic agent such as albuterol, given before aerobic exercise, usually completely blocks exercise-induced asthma. Sometimes this proves inadequate. Adding a few sprays of cromolyn can further decrease a child's difficulties with exercise.

Adding Oral Steroids

If short-acting bronchodilators such as albuterol are not adequate, you may sometimes have no choice but to give them oral steroids, and you should be happy they are available. These are the single most effective type of medication for asthma and should always, repeat, always, be given for severe asthma attacks. Any side effects are far less than the risk of an untreated severe attack. In fact, side effects from oral steroids when given for less than one to two weeks are usually minimal. The most common approach is to give five days of oral steroids and stop immediately. Sometimes physicians will decide that five days is not long enough, so they will continue these medications longer, often slowly weaning your child off. The most common side effects of these relatively short courses of oral steroids are increased appetite and perhaps mood changes, both of which stop as soon as you stop the medication. There really are no long-term side effects from a short course of oral steroids, though there is a long list of side effects with chronic use. Still, let's not forget how severe and dangerous asthma can be.

Before the development of inhaled steroids, a significant proportion of children with asthma were considered "steroid-dependent," meaning their asthma was only well controlled if they remained on oral steroids. Now that is unusual.

Key Point: *If your child is prescribed oral steroids, give them to her. Don't take a chance. Then ask if there is anything you can do differently next time. If you don't change the regimen, you may find yourself repeating this experience.*

Since oral steroids are prescribed for asthma all of the time, you would think there would be a consensus on dose and duration of treatment. But many physicians swear by different doses. How can this be? Partly because every child is different and responds differently. The art of medicine is in learning how to individualize for each patient.

I've noticed something that I don't believe has been scientifically studied. The less well a physician knows a patient, the more likely they are to prescribe steroids for acute asthma. This really makes sense, since it's better to be safe than sorry. As I'm sure you know there are very few physicians in solo practice left in the United States who take calls every night, and asthma always seems worse at night. (Actually, when I chose pulmonology, no one told me that all my patients would be sick at 3:45 A.M.) If you call your physician at night or on weekends because your child is wheezing or coughing, there is a better than even chance you will speak to a doctor who has never seen your child. They may prescribe oral steroids when your own doc might try to wait it out a little longer. If possible it is always better to speak to your child's own doctor during office hours. But don't be afraid to call even if you speak to a strange doctor.

If your child has required oral steroids before, you may feel very confident in making the decision yourself next time the same set of circumstances arises. Discuss with your physician the indications for starting oral steroids. In general, you should discuss this step with your physician, just to make sure you haven't forgotten anything.

Oral steroids are available as pills and liquids, but taste disgusting. Some kids don't seem to mind too much; some really can't stand these medications. The liquids taste somewhat better if they are refrigerated, but only slightly better. If your child can't swallow pills, remember that not all of the liquid preparations come in the same strength. Dosage mistakes can be made switching from one liquid to another. When given liquid medications, ask your doctor how many milligrams of medicine they are prescribing, not just how much volume of liquid (milliliters or ccs). Some liquid steroids contain 15 mg. per teaspoon, and some contain only 5 mg. per teaspoon. The classic oral steroids used for asthma are prednisone and its close relative, prednisolone. These both come in generic preparations and have been around a long time.

CURRENTLY AVAILABLE ORAL STEROIDS USED FOR ASTHMA

Generic Names	Brand Names
prednisone	Celestone
	Deltasone
prednisolone	Orapred
	Pediapred
	Prelone
dexamethasone	Decadron
hydrocortisone	Cortef
cortisone	Cortone

STEP #8:
Clarify how and when to start medicine, increase medicine, or decrease medicine.

This step is very important and frequently forgotten. If your child's asthma is triggered by tree pollen, you should expect to have to give medicines aggressively during the spring. If exercise is the culprit, then your child will be better able to participate in sports if a bronchodilator is given before athletic activities. If viral infections are a major trigger, then it is usually important to start medications at the onset of each cold. Many parents find it helpful to use a home peak-flow meter to assist them in these decisions.

WHAT YOU NEED TO KNOW ABOUT HOME PEAK-FLOW MONITORING

You may already have been given a peak-flow meter for home use. There are at least a dozen brands of peak-flow meters, and I don't think it matters which one you use. Most peak-flow meters are referred to as full-range models, meaning they are designed for any age child. Children younger than six or eight years of age are usually better served by a pediatric, or "low-flow," model. If your child starts out with a low-flow model, there will be a time when your child should graduate to a regular peak-flow meter.

What Is Peak Flow?

Peak flow—how hard a person can blow out, or the maximum flow of exhaled air your child can generate during exhalation—is a simple, easy way to quantify the severity of an asthma attack. As bronchospasm develops, the peak-flow (often abbreviated as PEF) measurement drops, often before any symptoms such as coughing or wheezing are present. As an asthma attack resolves, peak flow gradually returns to normal.

Should All Children with Asthma Have a Peak-Flow Meter?

No. The mother of an eight-month-old child asked me whether a peak-flow meter would help. I explained that peak flow takes a fair amount of effort, and that rarely can children perform the maneuver adequately until they are three or four years of age, sometimes not even until they are six or seven. She seemed genuinely disappointed, and then pulled a peak-flow meter she had received in the mail from her HMO out of her pocketbook! I guess some well-meaning person at her insurance company had decided that if their patients with asthma used peak-flow meters, perhaps they would get better and save the HMO lots of money. I suggested she save the meter for a few years.

Even if your child is old enough to use a peak-flow meter properly, not every child with asthma needs one. This should be a very individual decision. Peak-flow monitoring is time-consuming and many parents will decide it is not worth the bother.

What Then Is the Purpose of a Peak-Flow Meter?

The purpose of the peak-flow meter is to help you decide when to increase medicines, when you can safely decrease medicines, and when you need to seek medical attention. It is meant to be an early-warning device.

While peak-flow meters can help, remember that PEF can sometimes be either falsely high or falsely low. For instance, PEF may not drop before you or your child is already aware of a problem. And sometimes PEF can drop even when your child's asthma is not really that bad. Never let a peak-flow measurement replace your own instincts. If you believe your child needs medicine or medical attention, they do.

Does the Technique Used by My Child Matter?

Absolutely. Peak flow is very dependent on your child's effort. They need to practice taking in as big a breath as possible. After filling his or her lungs all the way, your child should insert the PEF meter past their teeth, and seal their lips around the mouthpiece. Then all they need to do is blow quickly into the meter, keeping their tongue out of the way. It is really much easier to show children how to measure their PEF properly than to describe the maneuver in words. Young children will do a better job standing up. In the past, doctors recommended that nose-clips be placed so air wouldn't leak out; however, more recent studies suggest that this really isn't worth the bother.

How Do I Know What My Child's Peak Flow Should Be?

Any healthcare provider who prescribes a peak-flow meter should also instruct you and your child on its use. At that time, she should estimate what your child's peak flow should be when he is well. You'll also learn what your child's range is on his own peak-flow meter. This is significant because just as home scales are most helpful on a relative basis, so, too, are peak-flow monitors. As your child grows, normal peak flow increases. Just as some perfectly healthy kids are tall and some are short, normal PEF varies quite a bit, even among kids of the same age, gender, and height. The best course is to determine your child's "personal best" and use that as your gauge.

How Can I Determine My Child's "Personal Best"?

First your child should measure his peak flow every day for a week or two while perfectly well. Even in healthy children, PEF may vary throughout the day, so try to obtain these measurements at the same time daily. The best time is usually first thing in the morning before any medications, as that tends to be the time of lowest peak flow. Have your child blow into the meter at least three times, and write down the best of the three. The highest measurement is, by definition, their peak flow.

Is the Goal to Keep My Child's Peak Flow Perfect?

Definitely not. That is neither necessary nor advisable. Your goal is to control your child's symptoms, not their peak flow. Most specialists recommend that a child's PEF be allowed to fluctuate approximately 20 percent lower than their personal best. This is known as your child's "green zone."

How Often Should I Have My Child Measure Her Peak Flow?

The more often you measure PEF, the more useful the information. Many national and international guidelines recommend that your child take these measurements at least once every day. To be honest, few kids want to do this, especially when they are doing well. And very few parents want to enforce this. However, if you want to be on top of the situation, it's worth the effort because by measuring it daily, you have the best chance of detecting a drop below your child's green zone.

How Can I Use My Child's Peak Flow to Help Manage Her Asthma?

After you have determined your child's personal best when well, the next step is to determine his Peak Flow Management Zones, as demonstrated in the figure on page 249: The green zone, usually above 80 percent of personal best, is where you want and hope your child will be most of the time. If your child's PEF drops into the yellow zone, it is time to either increase medications or add medications based on a personalized asthma action plan. As his asthma improves, peak flow will gradually return to the green zone, signaling that you can consider backing off some medications. The yellow zone is usually calculated to be between 50 and 80 percent of their personal best. If your child's PEF drops below 50 percent of their personal best—into the red zone—seek medical attention.

Peak Flow Management Zones

Personal Best	GREEN ZONE	Great!
80% of Personal Best	YELLOW ZONE	Do something
50% of Personal Best	RED ZONE	Contact your physician

Key Point: *These zones are just guidelines. Only over time can you learn how to apply changes in peak flow to your child's care.*

STEP #9:
Don't leave your doctor's office without a plan for emergencies.

Every patient should have a written Asthma Action Plan, giving parents a clear step-by-step sequence of what to do and when, based on symptoms. "Call the doctor" or "Go to the hospital" are not enough. My patients always have at least three steps: (1) What to do if he starts to cough or wheeze; (2) What to do if the first step proves inadequate; and (3) When to seek medical attention.

Many asthma specialists have elegant printed asthma plans, multicolored and easy to read. I guess I'm just too cheap. I tried using some preprinted plans but they seemed to limit me and cramp my style. So I give each patient a handwritten plan, which means that there is another step in the process . . . making sure they can read my handwriting!

This plan must be individualized and depends, in part, on your child's triggers. The first step usually involves giving your child a treatment with a short-acting beta-adrenergic agent such as albuterol. This may be given orally, with an inhaler preferably with a holding chamber, or via nebulizer.

The second step usually involves how frequently and how often this "rescue" medication can be repeated. In some children who are triggered by viral illnesses, adding an inhaled steroid or raising their dose may be part of the plan. Some physicians give their patients a prescription for an oral steroid such as prednisone or prednisolone, with directions on when to use it and how much to give. Some physicians prefer their patients to call before starting prednisone.

The reasons for contacting your physician vary, but probably will include significant drops in your child's peak flow, failure of the regimen to work adequately, or if you believe oral prednisone may be necessary. Obviously, when in doubt, always call.

Hang on to your plan and refer to it whenever your child is sick. Recently I met Cynthia in the emergency room. Six-year-old Cynthia had started wheezing two or three days before. She had been so well controlled on just cromolyn that she hadn't had any asthma symptoms in more than a year; so when she started to cough and complain of feeling tight in the chest, her mom had forgotten what to do. She found an old albuterol inhaler in the drawer, but it had long expired. Cynthia's mom increased the cromolyn from two puffs to four puffs, and from twice to three times a day. When that wasn't working, she started giving her four sprays of cromolyn every two to three hours through the night. Finally, after a terrible night of gasping for breath, Cynthia was brought to her local community hospital and then transferred to the medical center where I work. Imagine how Mom felt when reminded that cromolyn is of little value during an acute asthma attack?

STEP #10:
Plan follow-up visits.

No visit or phone call with your healthcare provider is complete without a clear follow-up plan. I believe strongly that some sort of routine follow-up visit schedule should be planned, even if your child is doing well. The frequency of visits should be specified, and most children need to be seen more than annually. History gets forgotten when the intervals are stretched, so I insist on at least every six months for my patients.

You also need to discuss which physician is primarily going to help you with making changes in the plan. Many patients have both a primary care provider and a specialist. Some patients have more than one specialist, e.g., an allergist and pulmonologist.

Key Point: *Discuss the issue of overlapping roles with your healthcare providers. Their job is to make your life easier, not harder.*

TAKE-HOME MESSAGES

- It's not the specific medicines that count, it's the goals.

- Clarify your goals and choose a regimen that makes sense to you.

- Always ask yourself if your regimen meets your needs. If not, change it.

- Decide on daily preventive therapy or therapy just as needed.

- Have a clear plan that includes both daily and as needed medications.

- Consider a peak-flow meter to help guide medication adjustments.

- Don't settle for poorly controlled asthma or side effects from medications.

FOURTEEN

Asthma Triggered by Allergens

Karen is an adorable six-year-old who won't talk to me. According to her mom, she's a nonstop talker at home or with friends, but for some reason she gets really shy around me. This makes it hard to ask her how she feels. She was referred to me because she would cough every day in kindergarten and go to the school nurse, and her mom would have to leave work and bring her home. This started soon after the school year began, and it continued for about four months before they came to see me. Her mother had taken her to her pediatrician three times, but whenever she was in the doctor's office, Karen never coughed and her chest always sounded perfect. She had no other symptoms, not even a stuffy nose, and looked and sounded perfectly healthy in my office.

Her mother and pediatrician were pretty sure Karen was just having trouble adjusting to school and the pressures that six-year-olds often feel. But to be 100 percent sure, she came to me for an evaluation. I measured her pulmonary function in the office, and the tests really looked pretty normal, but I had another idea. I asked her mom to bring her to my office directly after picking her up from school so I could repeat the measurement. Sure enough, she came in coughing and her breathing tests were significantly worse than they were before. To confirm that she really was having mild asthma at school, I then gave her albuterol, the most common fast-acting asthma medication, and ten minutes later, her pulmonary function was back to normal and her cough was gone.

So, what was going on? Clearly she was having a reaction to something at school. This was not in her head. Mom went into the classroom and noticed that the kids started each day by feeding and playing with a sweet little guinea pig named Max. The next day, Mom instructed Karen and Karen's teacher that she should stay away from Max. Sure enough, no cough. She still won't talk to me, though. Oh well.

For people with asthma, allergens are the most common trigger. Asthma is a condition in which the bronchial tubes overreact to substances that are inhaled and land directly on the air passages. Except for infants who sometimes wheeze because of cow's milk allergy, most kids with allergic asthma are triggered not by foods but by inhaled allergens: dust mites, pollens, mold spores, animal danders, even cockroaches.

Many families don't realize their child's mild morning cough is related to something to which she is allergic, and if they do make the connection, they are more likely to suspect the allergic reaction is to food.

The basic information about asthma management is covered in Chapter 13. There are some additional steps that will help reduce asthma by reducing allergies. This chapter will address what you need to know that is specific to allergy-induced asthma.

Recognizing That Allergies May Be a Factor

The nose is just another airway, not all that much different from the lower airways or bronchial tubes. Usually if the lower airways are sensitive to allergens (asthma), then so are the upper airways (hay fever).

How do you know if allergies are playing an important role in your own child's asthma? Sometimes it takes years for a pattern to become discernible, partly because some allergies develop over time and partly because the number of respiratory infections in young children often mask the symptoms of allergy. When I am evaluating a child for the first time for coughing or wheezing, I also want to know if there are signs of allergies:

1. Dry skin, or eczema
2. History of hives or other itchy rashes
3. History of bad reactions to any foods
   or medications
4. Snoring
5. Itchy eyes, particularly in the spring or fall
6. Chronic runny nose or sneezing, particularly
   in the morning

Next I assess whether there is a family history of allergies, particularly in the child's immediate family. It doesn't matter that much, but a completely negative family history makes allergies much less likely.

Key Point: *Children with asthma due to allergies almost always have other allergy symptoms, such as hay fever (allergic rhinitis).*

The next step is looking for patterns to your child's symptoms. The most common indoor allergen, for instance, is dust mites, those little creatures that like to hang out in your bed with you at night. Chronic sneezing and coughing in the morning is a strong indicator that such an allergy may exist, though you should also consider other indoor allergens such as mold spores or cockroaches.

Allergies to pollen tend to develop a bit later in life, so your school-age child may start sneezing and coughing each spring, and as a result, her asthma may become worse.

What Allergens Trigger Your Child's Asthma?

If your child's asthma is predominantly triggered by allergies, minimizing exposure is far preferable to medicating. Unfortunately, prevention is much more difficult and requires consistent effort over time. (See Chapter 8 for advice on minimizing allergens in the home environment.) The first step is to determine which allergens trigger your child's asthma, not always an easy task. In young children, frequent viral respiratory infections can confuse the issue—does she have a cold, or is she allergic to something? Allergic kids often have many allergies, so it is difficult to pinpoint which allergen is triggering asthma. Accurate allergy testing is critical.

Allergy tests aren't perfect, and only by combining tests with a careful history can allergies be accurately determined. A good allergist will rely on a combination of allergy testing and "mommy-testing." An observant parent who spends the most time with the child—whether it's Mom or Dad—will likely have a good hunch as to what the allergen is. If the sneezing occurs mainly on Mondays, the day the child spends the afternoons at Grandma's, the family should investigate that environment. Does Grandma have a cat? Is there a damp lower-floor recreation room where there may be mold? Does Grandma keep a lot of indoor plants? If your child was triggered by respiratory infections this winter, with no symptoms in between "colds," then it is unlikely that indoor allergens are important problems. If, however, you notice mild asthma symptoms cropping up in between infections, allergies should be suspected.

An allergy to a family pet can be difficult to prove, mainly because pet dander may have spread throughout your home (even when your pet is happily sleeping on the back porch), making it easy to notice that your child is allergic to something but hard to identify that something. That's when well-thought-out allergy testing must play a part.

Key Point: *What separates a good allergist*
              from a lousy one is the ability to
              consider all factors, including
              the geographical area, the season,
              and the parental "hunch" factor,
              and then run appropriate tests and
              interpret them properly.

Keep in mind that plenty of kids catch colds (viral infections) even in May and June. Generally, the way to distinguish between a cold and an allergy is to consider whether your child has loss of appetite, fatigue, fever, or body aches. If these additional symptoms are present, then you can rule out allergies. Allergies can cause a sore throat, rarely swollen glands, but not fever. Infections cause fever.

Daily Preventive Medicine or As Needed?

No parent wants their child to remain on daily medication, and it is perfectly appropriate to try to avoid that. As with asthma medications, think in the short term rather than the long term. What is best for your child for this season—daily preventive therapy or as needed? Next season you can make a new decision. If you can control your child's asthma symp-

toms by controlling their nasal symptoms with allergy medications such as antihistamines and nasal sprays, that's great.
Unfortunately, this approach often proves inadequate and
most kids with allergic asthma need a balance of both allergy
and asthma medications. Basically, the rule stands:

Key Point: *Use the least amount of medication
to control symptoms so they don't
affect your child's lifestyle.*

Parents sometimes forget that most kids with asthma are
triggered by both allergies and infections and that their child's
medical regimen usually must be altered somewhat depending on the situation. Allergy medicines may be adequate much
of the year, but asthma medications will be important during
viral respiratory illnesses.

Choosing a Daily Preventive Regimen

In Chapter 13, various options for controller medications
were presented. Here I'm going to focus on the pros and cons
of these medications for allergy-induced asthma.

Daily low-dose inhaled steroids are my first choice for
most children with allergic asthma. While most parents are
understandably anxious about risks, allergic asthma can usually be controlled with remarkably low doses—ones that I
truly believe are safe, certainly safer than chronic undertreated asthma.

Some parents feel strongly about starting with one of the
nonsteroidal anti-inflammatory medications, such as cromolyn (Intal) or nedocromil (Tilade), or one of the
leukotriene modifiers, zafirlukast (Accolate) or montelukast
(Singulair). Some kids can be controlled using these milder
medications alone, but most cannot. What often occurs is

that a child becomes sick despite one of these nonsteroidal medications, requiring the addition of oral steroids. If the goal is to use the lowest dose of steroids possible, you may be better off starting out with low doses of preventive steroids rather than repeatedly requiring higher doses when your child becomes ill.

Both leukotriene modifiers and long-acting beta agonists are important medications for the child with allergic asthma. If you are constantly forced to raise the dose of inhaled steroids, one or two of these should be added as so-called steroid-sparing agents. By mixing a couple of medicines together in what is hoped to be a synergistic way, you can often keep down the risks of any one of the drugs to essentially nonexistent. Again, these are complex decisions that need to be individualized for each child, season by season.

Which "Rescue" Medications Are Best?

Reliever medications are usually members of the family of drugs called short-acting beta-adrenergic agonists, discussed in detail in Chapter 13. Within this category, albuterol attached to a spacer or holding chamber is by far the most commonly prescribed. As mentioned in Chapter 13, there is nothing sacred about two puffs; many kids need and can safely be given more than that. With my patients, I am very comfortable increasing the number of sprays to as high as five to ten sprays if lower doses aren't adequate.

Plan for Emergencies

Allergic reactions can happen anywhere. Ask your doctor for written instructions about how to handle an emergency and give copies to baby-sitters, school nurses, camp nurses, grandparents, separated spouses . . . anyone who might need to refer to the plan. I have always been proud of the individualized plans I give to every parent, but not long ago I realized that I was leaving out a very important piece of information: the date. One mother confessed she was confused as to which emergency plan was current because she had saved all the plans the family had received from me over the years. While families would be advised to toss out copies of old plans when new ones arrive, I know that many people forget to do that, so her comments were a good lesson for me. Now I date every plan.

Plan for Follow-Up Visits

I have emphasized the importance of routine visits before. Kids change, and their needs change. If a regimen isn't working well, change it. If a child is doing extremely well, think about decreasing medications.

The frequency of appointments varies considerably depending on the age of your child, the frequency of symptoms, and to some degree your comfort level and your child's asthma specialist's personal style. Sometimes I suggest six months and parents urge three. Sometimes I suggest two months and parents were thinking about six months. Discuss the timing of appointments so that you're all in agreement. Sometimes particular environmental allergens that bother your child dictate the planning. If your child seems to always have trouble in October, then perhaps that's a good time to schedule your next appointment. Or better yet, see the doctor in September to make sure you have a plan to prevent trouble in October. Don't leave it open-ended. Schedule the next appointment before you leave the office.

TAKE-HOME MESSAGES

- Allergens are common triggers for asthma, so if you maintain some control over your child's allergies, you will also help keep her asthma under control.

- Noting a pattern in asthma attacks can also help point out the offending allergens.

- Parents and physicians must decide together whether your child needs daily or as-needed medications for both allergies and asthma.

- Always request an emergency plan.

- Plan on routine follow-up visits and before each visit, ask yourself: "Am I happy with the current plan? Is the regimen we are using meeting our needs?"

FIFTEEN

Asthma Triggered by Infections

Although allergens are the most common cause of chronic low-level mild coughing and wheezing, respiratory infections are the most common cause of severe asthma attacks, including those that bring children to the emergency room or require hospitalization. Young children, especially those in day care or school or who have older siblings, may have eight to twelve infections from September to June, often blurring into a chronic nightmare for their parents. The good news is many young children who cough or wheeze with each cold may actually stop having significant symptoms of asthma later.

In fact, asthma specialists argue amongst themselves about what to call the condition of infection-induced wheezing in young infants. Should we lump this into the general term, Asthma? Experts of adult asthma think of Asthma with a capital "A" as a chronic inflammatory condition going on in the lungs all of the time, and essentially always associated with allergies. Just as someone with high blood pressure can never expect to come off their blood pressure pills, it follows that people with asthma should expect to always require chronic preventive therapy.

In pediatrics, we are more likely to stop daily medication when the number of infections drops down to a manageable level, usually when the child reaches about five to seven years of age, assuming that allergies haven't increased to take their place.

Remember, it is okay for your child to cough some with a respiratory infection. You want to find a way to control the symptoms so any coughing or wheezing is mild, manageable, and most importantly, gone within a couple of weeks. The overall principles of the management of asthma have been reviewed in Chapter 13. Let's get even more specific about what to do when asthma is triggered by an infection.

Prevention of Respiratory Infections

If you want to keep your child from having asthma that is triggered by an infection, then the reasoning is simple: Keep your child from getting infections. Good luck! If you can prevent infection then EUREKA, you can throw away all of the asthma medications. You may be able to reduce infections for a time, but in the long run this is not really practical. In other words, you can run but you can't hide. Catching colds (viral infections) is as much a normal healthy part of childhood as learning how to walk, talk, or losing your baby teeth. All children have relatively immature immune systems and develop frequent infections. If you keep them in a bubble for a time you can reduce this, but the maturation of their immune system depends on getting kicked in the pants repeatedly with infections. Infants in day care exposed to lots of kids catch more infections through the winter than kids kept away from other young children. But eventually children who are isolated will get the required infections, albeit at a later stage.

I hasten to add that there are children who are very fragile, such as tiny premature infants and babies with chronic lung or heart diseases that may need protection until they are older and better able to handle infections. For otherwise healthy children, though, prevention of infections is probably not worth it. And now with so many moms working outside of the home, keeping your children away from other kids with runny noses is just not practical. So my vote: Try not to worry about it too much. Do what you gotta do.

Incidentally, the only practice that has been consistently proven to reduce the number of infections is good and frequent hand washing. If you teach your toddler to wash his hands after picking up every disgusting or dirty thing he sees (and may even put into his mouth just for fun), write to me. (I won't be sitting by the mailbox waiting.)

Types of Respiratory Infections and the Problem with Antibiotics

There are many kinds of germs that could infect your child, but children with normal immune systems usually have to deal with two big categories: bacteria and viruses. If your child should happen to develop something stranger, such as a fungal infection of the respiratory tract, they need a careful evaluation of their immune system.

The vast majority of respiratory infections are due to viruses, and we currently have very few antibiotics that help fight viral infections. Even the new medications that have come out designed for influenza, for instance, only help a little. So for most respiratory illnesses, antibiotics don't help.

One of the most confusing diagnoses is "bronchitis." Many physicians were trained that if they heard the sounds in your chest consistent with bronchitis, then antibiotics were appropriate. Actually, bronchitis in both kids and adults is usually triggered by viral infections, with the exception of smokers. That's when bacterial bronchitis requiring antibiotics becomes more common.

You notice I didn't say antibiotics are *never* helpful. Bacterial infections can occasionally trigger coughing and even wheezing on occasion, and sometimes antibiotics do help. We now understand, for instance, that even young children can develop bacterial infections of the upper respiratory tract including the sinuses, and that these infections do seem in some mysterious way to trigger asthma.

The real problem is we almost never can tell for sure which germ triggered your child's illness. So this leaves us with the nagging doubt that antibiotics might help.

So why not just give an antibiotic? Isn't that safer, since they may help? Unfortunately, this is not uniformly the best approach. The development of antibiotics is clearly one of the most dramatic and important advances in the last one hundred years. But, with constant usage, many bacteria are growing resistant to treatment. This is not a little theoretical problem; it's a really big problem and getting worse. Also, many children are developing allergic reactions to antibiotics. Not only does this mean they won't be able to use that antibiotic or any compound chemically related to it ever again, children have died from allergic reactions to antibiotics.

Key Point: *Be very cautious with antibiotics, and only ask for them or agree to give them to your child if there are no safer alternatives.*

Medicate for Asthma As Needed or Preventively?

If infections are your child's only important asthma trigger, you may be able to get away with using asthma medications only when they get sick if (a) they don't get sick very often, such as during the summer, or after a child is five or six years of age, and (b) if your as-needed plan adequately controls their asthma when they do get sick. As mentioned repeatedly, if they are triggered frequently and/or starting and stopping medicine isn't meeting your needs, you should consider a daily preventive approach.

All respiratory infections have the same natural history:
1. The "getting sick" phase
2. A middle "sick but stable" phase
3. The "getting better" phase

Key Point: *The key to success is to start medications or increase medications during that first "getting sick" phase so you can head the illness off at the pass.*

If you can stop symptoms from progressing to what you consider an unacceptable amount and hold tight until the illness resolves, you will be happy with your approach.

Key Point: *Don't assume the same preventive regimen will be adequate if you decide to just use medications as needed.*

One advantage of a preventive approach is that you may get by with considerably lower doses of medications, unlike the as-needed approach, which may require high doses for shorter periods of time.

Choosing Specific Controller Medications

Since most research has been done looking at chronic allergy-triggered asthma, there is little agreement on which medications work best for infections and at what dose. Many respiratory infections in young children, unfortunately, trigger significant coughing and wheezing despite any controller regimen. Inhaled steroids remain the number one choice. Some of the newer oral asthma medications such as Accolate or Singulair are very safe; however, it's really not clear if these medications are adequate for asthma triggered by respiratory infections. While chronic long-term use of oral steroids such as prednisone has the potential for very significant side effects, short courses of oral steroids (less than one or two weeks) have minimal risk and are often necessary. Some asthma experts are comfortable instructing parents to rely on oral steroids for each significant asthma exacerbation. In general, I believe that if your child is requiring frequent short bursts of oral steroids, another approach should be tried. My impression is that higher doses of inhaled steroids are usually required for bad viral infections rather than for controlling day-to-day allergy-induced asthma.

So if your child requires a preventive strategy, the trend in recent years has been to recommend a very low dose of inhaled steroids on a daily basis even when your child is well, and if need be, to abruptly double or even triple the dose during any viral exacerbations. I hope to see more scientific data on this approach in the near future.

For intermittent treatment, choose appropriate medications.

Start albuterol or one of the short-acting beta-agonists as soon as your child starts with asthma symptoms. The specifics about these medications were reviewed in Chapter 13. These medications do not make an infection go away faster, but often adequately control asthma symptoms during the infection. Generally speaking, the sooner you start the better. If you know that every time your child develops a runny nose for more than four hours they end up coughing or wheezing, there is no reason to wait, start your motors. If your child, especially when older, can actually get through some mild colds without significant chest symptoms, then you might wait for coughing. Try not to wait until full-blown wheezing.

As discussed in the overview chapter, home peak-flow monitoring can really help. Remembering the limitations mentioned previously, a significant decrease in peak-flow often but not always occurs before you are aware of any symptoms, particularly in older children. So if you see a drop, start your first-line medication. But never let an inexpensive little plastic gizmo replace your own parental instincts. If you feel your child needs medicine, give it. And please, don't wait for wheezing, start with coughing.

When do you stop medications? My usual advice is that it is safer to continue albuterol until there is no cough, no rattle, no congestion, no wheeze, completely perfect . . . and then wait at least a couple of days. Don't stop after just four hours of no coughing.

Key Point: *Particularly during the school*
              year when everyone is sick, get
              your child back to perfect before
              the next infection.

Consider additional medications if
beta-adrenergic agents prove inadequate.

Most national and international asthma guidelines for physicians only recommend short-acting medications such as albuterol for patients just taking intermittent medication. If that fails, the standard is oral steroids, usually for three to seven days. This may be changing.

Many asthma specialists including me have become convinced that immediately increasing the dose of inhaled steroids at the beginning of a respiratory infection will sometimes help control your child's symptoms until the virus has left the body. So the obvious question is, can your child get by just using inhaled steroids during each respiratory illness? There have been remarkably few studies examining this approach, yet many patients are doing just that, whether or not they tell their physicians. Perhaps if you promptly start inhaled steroids at the onset of a viral respiratory illness (runny nose, mild cough), you will adequately control your child's symptoms without oral steroids. Many asthma specialists are going along with this approach. Physicians need to commit to relying on good scientific evidence as a basis of their practice, and I urge academic asthma specialists to study this approach. In the meantime, let me tell you some of the things I have learned about "as needed" inhaled steroids:

- They have almost no chance of working unless you start early in the illness.
- If the infection accelerates very quickly, oral steroids really are necessary.
- Young children go from really well to really sick really fast. So they often need a preventive daily dose of inhaled steroids.
- This approach may help control wheezing and even chesty, productive coughing. However, a dry hacking cough remains, for me, the most difficult respiratory symptom to control.
- Low daily doses of inhaled steroids used to control allergic asthma often prove inadequate for respiratory infections. If you don't want your child on daily medication the whole school year, you usually need higher doses for the duration of each cold.

- When your child wheezes or complains of
  chest tightness with viral infections, don't
  just use inhaled steroids. Combine them
  with a bronchodilator such as albuterol.

Treatment with Cough and Cold Remedies

What about cold and cough remedies? Aren't you amazed by how many there are? I once tried to count them, and between prescription and nonprescription medicines, I lost track after about two hundred. And I didn't even count all of the natural, herbal, and homeopathic remedies out there. So what should you do?

Key Point: *Try to use the least amount of medicine possible. Less is more.*

The trend in the industry has been to combine all kinds of stuff together in the hopes of making it easy to control coughing, sneezing, nasal congestion, itching, pain, headache, etc. Soon we should see one of these multisymptom medications include something for the heartburn caused by all of the other ingredients.

Despite these caveats, I do sometimes recommend these kinds of medicines, but only carefully and with great thought. In fact, I pride myself on learning how to use cold remedies appropriately, and I suspect many physicians don't bother too much.

So here are my opinions, again with very little scientific evidence to back me up:

Key Point: *Like most pulmonologists, I don't like cough suppressants.*

"Cough" in the name of a preparation usually signifies an ingredient such as dextromethorphan, which suppresses coughing. If your child is coughing, that usually means there is something down in the airways trying to come up. If you suppress the cough, you may buy some sleep, but you may also slow the resolution of the illness and actually worsen the situation. There is a major exception to this rule: dry hacking nonproductive coughs from postnasal drip. However, if you hear phlegm in the cough, be wary of cough suppressants.

Key Point: *Expectorants seem like a good idea,*
but usually aren't worth the bother.

If suppressing the cough is a bad idea, then medications that loosen secretions and help your child to get that stuff up would seem to make sense. The problem is that the currently available products just don't seem to do much for chest congestion. At high doses, these medications may help, especially for sinus and nasal congestion, but again, not that much. You should think of asthma medications such as albuterol as the most effective expectorants currently available.

Key Point: *Decongestants can help nasal*
congestion and coughing from
postnasal drip, but must be used
carefully if your child has asthma.

The most common oral decongestant in the United States is pseudoephedrine, usually referred to by the common brand name, Sudafed. While drying up a runny nose and decreasing postnasal drip can be very helpful, if there is significant asthma or chest congestion I am concerned that any secretions in the chest will thicken. If you are certain that your child's asthma is under very good control, judicious use of decongestants can be comforting. But remember the rule: Less is more.

Key Point: *Old-fashioned first-generation*
antihistamines may help relieve the
symptoms of an upper-respiratory-
tract infection, but the newer
allergy preparations, such as
Allegra, Clarinex, Clariten, and
Zyrtec, really won't help much.

When my kids were young, our favorite medicine at home was Dimetapp elixir. This is a classic combination of a first-generation antihistamine and a decongestant. There are many medicines like this and every family and pediatrician learns to use a few of these for the symptoms of a cold. They can really help. Once again, I worry about this kind of stuff worsening any asthma component of the illness. Discuss this carefully with your child's doctor, and also be sure to keep any chest congestion under control.

As Always, Plan for Emergencies

Viral respiratory infections are a normal part of childhood. Expect them to occur and make sure you are clear on what to do next time your child is ill. Then be sure you know what to add if that first approach isn't cutting it. Finally, make sure you are clear on what to do if your first two steps aren't working. While it is a good goal to try and avoid oral steroids such as prednisone, the reality is that some of the time you may have no choice. It is important to discuss with your child's doctor how to decide when to start oral steroids, and what dose is appropriate. It is also important to discuss how often you can safely give your child short-acting bronchodilators, such as albuterol. Finally, it is important to know when it is time to call for help or go to the nearest emergency room.

Plan for Follow-Up Visits

As you've read, there is simply too much to review with your child's physician at a yearly routine "well-child visit" to have a proper discussion about asthma. Separate visits just to handle this subject are almost essential, except perhaps for the mildest patients. The frequency of these routine visits can vary considerably, depending on the personal style of your child's asthma doctor, your own comfort level, the age of your child, and the number of respiratory infections he has.

Key Point: *You can't stop kids from getting sick, but you should be able to control their asthma so they can catch a cold without it always "going to their chest."*

TAKE-HOME MESSAGES

- Respiratory infections are the most common trigger for severe asthma attacks.

- When your child has an infection, discuss with your doctor temporary increases in her asthma medications.

- Be sure your doctor provides you with an emergency plan.

- If the treatment plan isn't working, ask for a new plan. There are many, many possibilities out there, and it may take a few visits to find the right one for your child.

- Keep up with your follow-up visits. Be prepared for the next cold.

SIXTEEN

Asthma Triggered by Exercise

When parents hear of exercise-induced asthma or "EIA," most imagine the worst-case scenario: A running child collapses with severe wheezing. Everyone stops what they're doing, an ambulance is called, and your child is whisked away for treatment, never again permitted to participate in sports. Fortunately, this type of severe reaction is extremely rare, though milder forms of exercise-induced bronchospasm (asthma) are very common. Under certain conditions, almost anyone may develop spasm of the muscles that encircle our bronchial tubes (our airways) during exercise. It can occur in children who are in perfect health as well as those who have already been diagnosed with asthma.

Exercise-induced bronchospasm does not occur when someone simply runs up the stairs; it requires more exertion. (If your child seems short of breath with brief periods of exercise, look for other reasons.) For exercise to trigger bronchospasm, a person needs to be exercising hard, huffing and puffing for about four to six minutes. The amount of bronchospasm that develops is almost directly related to the amount of air per minute that is being moved in and out of your lungs. The harder the exercise, the more air goes in and out of the lungs; therefore, the more intense the reaction. Most kids breathe in between three and six liters of air per minute while relaxing in front of the TV. During an intense soccer game, those same children may be breathing in thirty to sixty liters of air per minute, or even more.

Mild symptoms may go unrecognized. There may be no obvious wheezing, and sometimes not even coughing. Kids frequently complain of just feeling tired, short of breath, or having vague chest discomfort. However, if symptoms are more pronounced, a child may wheeze, cough, and have difficulty breathing; some describe outright chest pain. The most common reason for chest pain in teenagers referred to cardiologists has nothing to do with their heart, but is, in fact, mild bronchospasm. Those with mild symptoms often assume that they are simply out of shape or, even worse, nonathletic. This perception of poor athletic ability may lead to a sedentary lifestyle and can be tough on a child's self-image, particularly since sports are so intrinsic to our modern culture. Many children gradually turn away from sports and exercise because of unrecognized or undertreated exercise-induced asthma.

MAJOR SYMPTOMS OF
EXERCISE-INDUCED ASTHMA
- Wheezing
- Shortness of breath
- Chest tightness
- Cough (after sports or coming in
  from playing outside)
- Chest congestion
- Chest pain or discomfort

MORE SUBTLE SIGNS OF
EXERCISE-INDUCED ASTHMA
- Feels out of shape or winded
- Tires easily

- Displays lack of energy
- Has problems while running but not while swimming
- Is unable to keep up with friends when running or playing
- Is unable to run five minutes without stopping
- Becomes dizzy after exercise
- Develops frequent stomachaches
- Clears throat frequently

Quick Check: Action Plan for Exercise-Induced Asthma

When to Call Your Doctor

If your child has to stop exercising or has any bothersome symptoms, call your doctor and discuss a change in medications. Don't settle for uncontrolled symptoms.

When to Seek Immediate Medical Attention

Your instincts won't fail you. If your child is breathing hard or constantly coughs even after treatment, speak to a physician. If there is any change in alertness or she can't speak, consider calling for emergency help (911).

Many but not all children can recognize a pattern to their exercise-induced asthma. The first early phase is the most severe. Usually symptoms occur after five to fifteen minutes of exercise and may worsen even after exercise has ended, gradually resolving on their own after about thirty to sixty minutes. About half of all patients then experience a "refractory period" during which they feel fairly well. After this thirty-to-ninety minute grace period, bronchospasm may recur, even twelve to sixteen hours later, lasting for up to twenty-four hours.

Addressing the Condition
Can Prevent Emergencies

Exercise-induced asthma is not usually dangerous. Kids can and often do run right through the spasm, and sometimes it will let up on its own. Very rarely, exercise triggers life-threatening bronchospasm, and this usually occurs in someone who has already had significant narrowing of the bronchial tubes before they start exercising. That's one reason why you should make sure your child's asthma is well controlled before exercise.

Optimizing lung function is one key to reducing the likelihood of EIA. Doctors automatically listen for phlegm and "rattly" breathing, which is a good start to checking lung function. In addition, some pediatricians and all asthma specialists have equipment to accurately measure your child's pulmonary function. Remember, when well, your child's lung function should be normal or very close to it.

I am often asked what limitations should be placed on children who sometimes experience EIA, and parents are surprised when I rarely set limits—with one exception:

Key Point: *Children who are having difficulty*
breathing or are already wheezing
should not participate in exercise
until their breathing difficulties
are resolved.

Otherwise, I encourage my patients to participate in almost every activity in which they are interested. There is no reason why they can't be in the Olympics, and it's important that children understand this. In fact, at least one in six athletes at the 1996 Olympic Games had a history of asthma, and about 10 percent had active asthma requiring medications during the games. Too many people with asthma grow up with a sedentary lifestyle—an unnecessary and unhealthy way of life.

If your child is considering high-level competitive sports, remember that while prescription asthma medications are approved by most organizations sponsoring sports competitions, many medications are not, including certain cold and cough remedies.

Be reassured that there should be little reason for your child to sit out any activities, whether in gym, during recess, at summer camp, or during organized sports.

Raymond's EIA

An experience with my own son's soccer team presented to me one of my most memorable encounters with a child who had exercise-induced asthma. Nine-year-old Raymond was an incredible athlete. Wherever the ball was, so was Raymond. My son, Sam, taking after me, tended to hang back, trying to stay out of trouble, but Raymond loved to get into the thick of things. When Raymond showed up, the team won. If Raymond missed a game, we were doomed. But then one particular Sunday, Raymond didn't seem to be on his game. He was phoning it in. His father was distinctly upset, yelling and screaming from the sidelines, "Raymond, come on!" "Wake up!" "Raymond, What the h——'s the matter with you?" During halftime, I happened to be standing next to Raymond, and *Raymond was wheezing!* Quietly, but unequivocally, he was wheezing; and no one knew it. His father didn't know it, Raymond didn't know it. No one realized what was happening.

So now I had a dilemma. There was no immediate need to become involved, most kids can play right through exercise-induced asthma. Generally I prefer to remain anonymous at these soccer games, and to tell you the truth, Raymond's father looked a little scary to me. On the other hand, the boy was getting a lot of heat from his dad for not playing with his usual zeal. What to do?

I came up with what I thought was a brilliant plan. I sent my wife. I said to Donna, "Just go over there and mention (gently) to Raymond's dad that you couldn't help notice that Raymond was wheezing." And, amazingly, it worked. Raymond's dad turned out to be a nice guy; he was genuinely surprised and quite concerned. Donna suggested he speak to Raymond's pediatrician about it on Monday.

But the story didn't end there. The very next day a local pediatrician called and asked me to squeeze in some kid named Raymond as soon as possible. Well, *this was Raymond,* and next Sunday was another soccer game, so I found time for him ASAP. A simple inhaler taken fifteen minutes before each game worked perfectly. Raymond was back to being as aggressive and amazing as ever and our soccer team won again that Sunday.

By the way, Raymond's dad wasn't the only parent to miss EIA in his own child. My son had a mild croupy cough a few times as a young child and would occasionally complain of feeling tight in the chest, but somehow I kept forgetting that he might benefit from an inhaler before those games. By this time, many people in my small town were aware of my profession, so imagine my embarrassment when he yelled out in the middle of a game, "Daddy! I'm wheezing!"

The Causes of Exercise-Induced Asthma

Until the mid-1970s, we understood very little about how exercise triggers asthma. Back then, a number of scientists asked a simple question: "Does everyone with asthma respond negatively to exercise, and if not, why not?" For some reason the fraction of people with asthma who wheezed with exercise varied from one research study to another, and no one knew why. It did seem that exercise in cold, dry air, such as running in the winter, was more likely to trigger asthma than exercising in warm, humid air, such as swimming in the summer.

A series of breakthrough studies, predominantly designed and performed by a group of Harvard scientists led by Dr. Regis McFadden, involved triggering exercise-induced asthma in adult volunteers and measuring the effects of changing the air they breathed. When volunteers rode an exercise bike while breathing specially conditioned air from a reservoir bag, the greatest bronchospasm occurred when the air was very cold and dry. Adults with a clear history of exercise-induced asthma often developed no bronchospasm at all when their inhaled air was warmed to body temperature and fully humidified, just like the air within their lungs. In other words, when there was no difference at all between the conditions of the air in their lungs and the inhaled air, exercise-induced asthma did not occur, regardless of how hard the volunteers exercised. (Of course this is an experimental finding in a laboratory where the inhaled air was maintained at 98.6° Fahrenheit and 100 percent humidity. In the real word, children can still develop asthma while exercising in warm humid air, though it is less likely.)

My colleagues and I were very excited about these studies in adults. We adapted this work to children and showed that almost all asthmatic children would develop symptoms after breathing cold dry air hard and fast for about four minutes, even without exercise. These studies led us to appreciate the importance of cooling and drying the bronchial tubes (airways) during exercise.

How Exercise Triggers Asthma

Vigorous exercise

  ↓

    Increased oxygen demand

      ↓

        Increased rate and depth of breathing

          ↓

            Airway cooling and drying

              ↓

                Release of chemicals from cells within the airways

                  ↓

                    Narrowing of the airways

Other Factors That Contribute to EIA

There are a variety of additional factors that make exercise-induced asthma worse or more likely to occur. This is known as the "double-whammy." A long list of inhaled triggers, including allergens, pollutants, and respiratory infections, stimulate the airways, increasing their sensitivity to exercise. Some of these, like cigarette smoke and known food allergens, can be avoided, but most are unfortunately part of modern life.

Factors That Contribute to Exercise-Induced Asthma
- Cold air
- Low humidity
- Airborne particles and pollutants (especially ozone, nitrogen dioxide, and sulfur dioxide)
- Inhaled allergens
- Irritants (smoke, cosmetics, art supplies)
- Car and truck exhaust
- Respiratory infections
- Fatigue
- Emotional stress

Children's Lifestyles and What Triggers EIA

You now see that if the air is cold and dry enough and exercise requires sufficient huffing and puffing, mild narrowing of the bronchial tubes can occur in anyone. Parents usually do not notice any difficulty with exercise until their child is between five and eight years old, when kids begin joining local soccer teams and are encouraged to run hard enough and long enough to develop bronchospasm. (Problems almost never occur in this age group during baseball or swimming seasons.) Eight- to ten-year-olds often play very hard during recess, so some kids begin to have symptoms during these years. Difficulties during physical education classes are more likely to occur during the middle school years, when physical education teachers expect a higher level of aerobic activity. The infamous mile run may be the first time a child notices a significant problem with breathing during gym.

By high school, organized competitive sports become the major challenges. EIA occurs commonly in teenagers participating in track, football, hockey, basketball, and tennis. However, the problem is not limited to these sports. I have also seen kids have difficulty with swimming, cheerleading, tumbling, and all sorts of dancing.

Because short sprints rarely trigger asthma, practices for basketball, track, football, and hockey are much more likely to cause trouble than the actual games. Downhill skiing rarely causes a problem because few participants have to work that hard. Despite the surrounding warm air, swimming at this level can trigger asthma, though problems are more likely to occur during practices or long-distance events.

Until recently, many physical education teachers and coaches were confused by exercise-induced asthma, uncertain whether kids were just faking it. Fortunately, most now understand how common these conditions are, how to design an exercise program to minimize difficulties, and what to do if an attack occurs.

Managing EIA

Actions can be taken to minimize or eliminate exercise-induced bronchospasm:

- Improve physical conditioning
- Decrease nasal congestion
- Avoid environmental irritants
- Warm up adequately
- Avoid foods to which you are sensitive
- Allow time for adequate cool-down
- Use appropriate medications

The first step is to keep your child active and exercising year-round so that her body is in good condition. The better shape you are in, the farther you can run before you start breathing hard—a crucial factor in triggering a reaction.

Many parents assume their kids are in good shape when they really aren't. Ask any professional athlete and they will tell you that a single week without aerobic exercise can lead to de-conditioning. Many kids go months between athletic seasons without frequent exercise. Splashing around the pool doesn't do it. Softball doesn't do it. Kids who are prone to exercise-induced bronchospasm should be encouraged to maintain a regimen of at least three sessions a week of aerobic exercise (I mean real huffing and puffing), each lasting for at least twenty minutes.

To avoid triggering bronchospasm, experienced coaches and gym teachers have learned the value of starting the season with a series of short sprints. Warm-up exercises and adequate cool-down periods are very important. Warm up may include walking or other low-level activities, stretching exercises, and running in place for two or three brief (thirty-second) periods about sixty seconds apart. Cool-down should last ten minutes or more.

Key Point: *Nasal congestion will make exercise-induced bronchospasm worse.*

The next step in EIA management is to consider the nose. The oft-ignored nose fulfills a very important role: Its job is to warm, humidify, and filter the air we breathe. Coaches often recommend that athletes practice breathing in through their noses and out through their mouths. If the nose is clear enough to breathe through during exercise, a child will not develop bronchospasm. There are many approaches to clearing the nasal passages, but the most common methods involve nose sprays. There are literally dozens of choices, both over-the-counter and prescription. And sometimes just a nice soft handkerchief is all that is needed.

Exercise-induced asthma can often be treated successfully by your general pediatrician or family physician. However, if you are concerned that your child is having more symptoms than you want, if the medications (see below) don't seem to be working, or if your child has had a low-level chronic cough for months at a time, even when well, then consider an evaluation by a specialist.

Medicines That Help

The goal of medication is to completely control exercise-induced bronchospasm so kids can participate in all activities. Side effects from medications are unacceptable.

No one medication is right for all kids. Everyone responds differently to various prescriptions, so it is important to work with your doctor to learn what is best for your child. The task of the medical professional is to assess the situation and through trial and error find what works for your child. Express your goals and the goals of your child. One of my patients loved Irish step-dancing, an extremely aerobic activity that entails hard-core huffing and puffing for three or four hours per session. Like most kids, my patient wanted to make it through practice uninterrupted, so we experimented with some of the newer long-acting medications and found one that worked for her. Had I assumed that the request for something "to help my daughter get through dance class" meant one hour of ballet, I would have not been providing the medication she needed.

Proper timing of medication is very important, and the challenge is to establish a schedule that works and minimizes any interruption in lifestyle. The ideal plan is one that doesn't require a child to go to the nurse for medication during the day; youngsters don't take well to having to do something different from what their friends are doing. One mother was frustrated with her thirteen-year-old, who never liked to go to the school nurse before lunch for his inhaler. It turned out that he had a perfectly good reason: If he was even five minutes late for lunch, he wouldn't get a seat at the same table as his friends.

Guidelines for Particular Forms of Exercise

Below are some suggestions for handling various situations. These are guidelines only, and specific medication selection must be worked out with your child's doctor. Details about all of these medications can be found in Chapter 13.

Sports

Most kids simply need to take a short-acting inhaler, most often two to four sprays, before a game or practice. By far the most commonly prescribed medication is albuterol, which is available in generic form as well as two common brands, Ventolin and Proventil. Because albuterol doesn't work immediately, this medication should optimally be inhaled at least ten to fifteen minutes before running. This schedule is usually not too difficult to work out for sports after school, in the evenings, or during the weekend.

Parents should discuss the situation with their child's physician after treatment has been tried a few times, or call immediately if severe breathing problems develop. A child should have no chest tightness, cough, or discomfort during or after exercise. If symptoms are not completely controlled, the problem may lie with faulty inhaling technique. Although they are bulky, spacer devices or holding chambers really help, and I urge their use for all standard metered-dose inhalers. Unfortunately, many kids find it inconvenient to carry a holding chamber with them to sporting events.

Inhaler technology is gradually improving, and some of the new inhalers do not require a spacer device. One such inhaler, Maxair Autohaler, is breath-activated and therefore very convenient for pretreatment before exercise. The active ingredient is pirbuterol, which is almost identical to albuterol. However, these newer breath-activated inhalers do require a different inhalation technique then recommended for standard inhalers with or without spacer devices. It is very important that proper technique be carefully taught and reviewed periodically. Kids less than six to eight years of age may not be able to completely benefit from these inhalers.

When prescribing an inhaler for exercise-induced bronchospasm, one of the unfortunate habits physicians fall into is limiting patients to only two sprays. While that dose may be adequate, some children may need three or four sprays of albuterol to completely block bronchospasm. This increased dosage is usually safe, but check with your physician. Sometimes more than one medication may be required. Cromolyn (Intal), nedocromil (Tilade), and montelukast (Singulair) can also help prevent EIA.

PHYSICAL EDUCATION CLASS

It may be difficult to know whether a child needs medication before a physical education class. Most kids will only need something for those occasional activities likely to trigger asthma, such as basketball or running outside in the cool air. Many other gym activities such as tumbling or volleyball are not a problem, especially if they are held indoors. If it is possible to know what is on the schedule, then parents can make that decision day to day. If the schedule is not certain, I recommend parents talk to the gym teacher. Most will be more than glad to see that your child receives their medications on the days they believe it appropriate. Since exercise-induced asthma is rarely severe, it is okay to let children with asthma try activities first to see how it goes. All children should feel free to participate in all activities without parent or child feeling fearful.

If medication is needed, the same short-acting medications discussed above, given ten or fifteen minutes before gym class, usually work well. The key is to adjust the timing of the medication depending on when the class is held. If class is within an hour or two of the start of school in the morning, then the simplest approach may be to take albuterol or pirbuterol before leaving for school. If class is later in the day, students may have to take their inhalers at school, usually just for the occasional highly aerobic activity like the mile run—which triggers dozens of referrals to our practice every year. Remember that the effect of albuterol wears off in a few hours. If it is not easy for kids to use an inhaler at school, then it may be worth discussing a long-acting medication to be taken before leaving home in the morning (see below).

RECESS

Recess is very important for many kids, serving as an welcome break in the day and an important social event. Many kids run around like maniacs. This is a great outlet for pent-up energy. Going to a nurse, taking an inhaler, and waiting fifteen minutes may not work for the school child who is desperate to get outside for what may only last fifteen or twenty minutes.

I hate to see kids unable to play with abandon. If your child is having trouble during recess and can't fit a short-acting inhaler into his or her schedule, talk to your doctor about a prescription for a long-acting medication in the morning. There are a variety of choices, each with their own advantages and disadvantages. Most are chemical cousins of albuterol, usually giving protection from exercise-induced bronchospasm for eight to twelve hours, and are available in both inhaled and pill form. The two long-acting inhalers available in the United States are Serevent (salmeterol) and Foradil (formoterol). Long-acting pills include Volmax or Proventil Repetabs (both time-released pill versions of albuterol), Singulair (montelukast), which comes in chewable and regular pill forms, and Accolate (zafirlukast). These last two are not related to albuterol and work by a very different mechanism.

SUMMER CAMP

Controlling exercise-induced bronchospasm at summer camp presents special challenges. Fortunately, most summer experiences take place during warm weather, so exercise is less likely to cause trouble. However, even then, highly athletic kids who go to intensive sports camps sometimes have difficulty.

If your child is attending sleep-away camp, it is important to have a clear written plan specific for that camp, including any routine medications as well as what to do for any symptoms (see Chapter 12). The last thing kids want to do during camp is leave their friends and wait in line at the nurse's office, so long-acting medications, given once or twice a day, are much more likely to actually be taken. In my experience, it is best to be flexible and to move the timing around so that medications are taken at mealtimes.

EIA AND ATHLETIC PROWESS

Sometimes a patient will be very disheartened by a diagnosis of EIA, fearing that if she has this condition, she'll have to drop her dream of being a great athlete. This often leads me to tell families about Jake, a tall and handsome high school student who came to see me. Jake was a serious long-distance runner, very competitive, maybe even thinking about the Olympics someday, and his parents were pretty intensely interested in this possibility. But after running fifteen or twenty miles, he would start to develop difficulty breathing. No cough, no wheeze that he knew of, just not feeling right. His parents had taken him to another pulmonologist, who suggested an exercise test to see what was going on. He completed a standard ten- to fifteen-minute exercise test and his lung function remained perfect, in fact better than perfect. So that doc sat down with Jake's parents and advised them to back off. He felt there was nothing wrong with their son, they were just pushing him too hard. He told them to stop being so competitive.

But they didn't buy that, so they came to see me. I decided to meet Jake at the exercise lab and see for myself what was going on. First, the lab tech measured his lung function and set him up on the treadmill. This kid was awesome. We cranked up that treadmill to its highest speed and greatest elevation; twenty minutes went by and he wasn't even breaking a sweat. His heart rate was still slow and steady. I was starting to gasp just watching him. Then, after about forty minutes, right before I was ready to give up, when I thought the poor treadmill might just collapse, he opened his mouth and started to huff and puff. Sure enough, four minutes later Jake was wheezing. Actual wheezing. Incredible. If your son or daughter is concerned about being diagnosed with EIA, share this story about Jake. Even the amazing athletes can have asthma.

Controlling Exercise-Induced Asthma

Is your child having any
trouble at all during or
after aerobic exercise?   NO ➡ Good. You get to worry
                                                about something else.

YES ⬇
Is your child already
known to have asthma?   NO ➡ Check with your child's
                                                doctor to see if the problem
                                                is EIA or some other reason
                                                for exercise intolerance.

YES ⬇
Is your child's asthma well
controlled before exercise?   NO ➡ Consider changes in base-
                                                line medications.

YES ⬇

Is your child's nose
chronically stuffed?   NO ➡ Consider evaluation
                                                   and prevention of nasal
                                                   congestion.

YES ⬇
Is your child's physical
conditioning what it
should be?   NO ➡ Encourage regular
                                                   aerobic exercise during off
                                                   seasons.

YES ⬇
Is your child receiving an
appropriate medication?   NO ➡ Remember, not all
                                                   medications for asthma pre-
                                                   vent exercise-induced
                                                   asthma.

YES ⬇
Is your child taking the
medication at the appropriate
time?   NO ➡ Each inhaler has a
                                                   different onset of
                                                   action. Check if your timing
                                                   is correct.

YES ⬇
Is your child's inhalation
technique correct? Does she
need a "spacer"?   NO ➡ Many children as
                                                   well as adults don't
                                                   inhale properly. Some re-
                                                   quire different
                                                   techniques.

YES ⬇

Is your child's exercise-
induced asthma now
completely controlled?   NO ➡ Consider a reevaluation by
                                               your physician or a special-
                                               ist.

YES ⬇

Great job! Remember, just when you have kids figured out, they change.

Exercise-induced bronchospasm can and should be completely controlled. Somewhere out there is a combination of
medications that works well for every child and doesn't cause
significant side effects. The trick is to find it. It is well worth
the effort.

TAKE-HOME MESSAGES

- Develop and encourage a regular physical
  conditioning program for your child even
  during the off season.

- Consider whether there is nasal congestion.
  A chronically stuffy nose due to allergies or
  other causes clearly worsens exercise-induced
  bronchospasm. There are almost countless
  medications and approaches to nasal congestion.
  Finding a successful approach can be tough,
  but it is well worth the effort.

- Be sure your child is breathing well going into an exercise activity. That means at a minimum, no cough, no phlegm, no rattling. Many kids as well as adults walk around partially bronchospastic, leaving little reserve for any further airway narrowing that may occur with exercise.

- If your child is already using an inhaler and still having symptoms, reevaluate timing, dose, and inhalation technique. Many kids do not allow sufficient time between their inhalers and actual exercise. Or there may be too many hours between medications and exercise. Most kids will find a spacer device or holding chamber very helpful for improving the protective effect of commonly prescribed inhalers (see Chapter 13). Sometimes patients need a dosage adjustment or the regimen needs to be changed. One medication may not always be adequate, two may be required.

- If simple medications do not solve the problem, remember there are a variety of rare explanations for chest pain, cough, chest tightness, or shortness of breath with exercise. Ask your doctor what else might be causing your child's symptoms.

PART FIVE:

ALLERGY ACTION PLAN: MEDICATION AND TREATMENT

SEVENTEEN

Allergic Rhinitis
(Nasal Allergies) and
Allergic Conjunctivitis
(Eye Allergies)

This chapter is dear to my heart, since I have allergic rhinitis and my nose is congested just about every day of my life. For some reason, patients find this very amusing. "You don't sound too good, Doc," they chide me. And when I sheepishly admit the reason I'm so stuffed up is because I forgot to take my allergy medicines, teenagers and their parents share a happy moment, relieved to know that even Dr. Dozor forgets to do what he is supposed to do. I have developed a very practical philosophy for myself, and it seems applicable to most of my patients.

Like anyone else, I don't like taking too much medication, but it is incredibly embarrassing to have a major sneezing attack in front of my patients. It's even more embarrassing to have to pull out a less than pristine handkerchief and blow my nose. So, when I decide what medications to take, at a minimum I try to prevent these major storms and I settle for sounding stuffy—that's acceptable to me.

Hay Fever: More Than an Annoyance

Though hay fever (allergic rhinitis) is often viewed as a mild annoyance, there is nothing minor about it to the child who is sneezing and has a runny nose, itchy eyes, congestion, and a sore throat from postnasal drip.

Rather than schedule a doctor's appointment, parents often reach for over-the-counter medications, but these are far from harmless. They may produce significant side effects including drowsiness (not good for the classroom), stomach distress, and irritability. In addition, overusing simple decongestant nasal sprays may create a condition known as "nasal rebound," where the spray actually creates more congestion by causing the mucous membranes of the nose to swell.

Many people mistakenly believe the symptoms of allergic rhinitis are limited to the nose. In fact, chronic nasal congestion causes many secondary effects. When your nose is obstructed, you can't sleep as well and can't smell as well. People with chronic nasal congestion are prone to headaches and recurrent sinusitis. Families frequently don't connect headaches with allergies, so sometimes children suffer for a long time without realizing that treating their allergies will help their headaches go away. Young children are particularly prone to repeated ear infections when they have allergies. Chronic mouth breathing leads to sore throats, hoarseness, and shortness of breath with even brief exertion, such as simply running up the stairs. Nasal congestion can also make exercise-induced asthma worse.

When good control of a child's hay fever is achieved, parents often notice significant improvements in mood, attention span, and general spirits, as their child can breathe quietly and easily—certainly a family goal worth shooting for.

Management of Allergic Rhinitis

Hay fever symptoms can be safely and effectively controlled.

MANAGING ALLERGIC RHINITIS

Identify your child's specific allergens.

↓

Minimize exposure without substantially
affecting lifestyle.

↓

Clarify your goals for your child's treatment.

↓

Plan your treatment approach for each
season: "preventive" vs. "as needed"
medications.

↓

Decide on oral vs. topical medications,
or both.

↓

Consider allergy shots
(immunotherapy).

↓

Be alert to the complications
of hay fever.

↓

Optimize therapy by
continually reevaluating the
medical approach.

Identify Your Child's Specific Allergens

Symptoms of hay fever (sneezing, itching, nasal congestion, morning cough, headaches, etc.) are usually due to inhaled allergens that land on the surfaces of your child's eyes, nose, and throat. (Foods do not cause hay fever.) If your child starts having coldlike symptoms in late March or early April, the hay fever season has probably begun. Most local papers, some radio stations, and the TV weather person have started giving pollen and mold spore reports. By paying attention to which counts are high, you'll begin to identify your child's most likely allergens. Since leafing trees are a sign of spring, those who are allergic to tree pollen are generally the early sufferers. Ragweed pollinates in the fall, so that may be a clue for you.

If this is your first visit to the doctor with a list of questions concerning allergies, refer to Chapter 3. It provides additional information on how to recognize which allergens may be playing a significant role in your child's symptoms.

Minimize Exposure Without Substantially Affecting Lifestyle

Indoor allergens such as dust mites and mold spores are much easier to mitigate than outdoor allergens, but there are still worthwhile measures to take to minimize exposure. For example, spring bouquets are fun to have in the house—if no one in the family has allergies. If someone sends you a beautiful arrangement of flowers, place the flowers in a room where allergic family members are least likely to encounter them. A garden bouquet brought in to the teacher really isn't a kindness for many kids in the class. As discussed in Chapter 10, you might also request that teachers keep blooming plants and flowers out of the classroom. And when Grandma visits, take her to the botanical gardens on your own when the kids are in school. Check pollen reports on the web or local newspaper to help plan outdoor activities. Keep your doors and windows closed and use air-conditioning during your child's worst season. Air-conditioning also reduces the level of humidity in your home, and this will help reduce both mold and dust mite allergen concentrations. Keep in mind that exposure to irritants such as cigarette smoke will worsen your child's hay fever.

If your child with allergic rhinitis still has significant symptoms despite preventive measures, then use medications so she can feel normal and participate in all of the fun things that make childhood so special.

Clarify Your Goals for Your Child's Treatment

Your child's hay fever should not interfere with her lifestyle. This varies from child to child, but it doesn't mean that your child can't have a stuffy nose or sneeze occasionally. I've had a stuffy nose since 1968! Waking up unrested is bad; having headaches from sneezing is no good; snoring to the point of developing sleep apnea is unacceptable. Your child should be able to play on the playground or be on a baseball team. Controlling hay fever may help keep asthma or sinusitis at bay.

Don't settle for side effects from medications. One child may feel just fine with a particular antihistamine, and another child of the same age will fall asleep in the middle of the day when given the same exact dose. Drowsiness may improve over time, but try to find medications that don't make your child sleepy at all. Sometimes the side effects are worse than the symptoms you are trying to control.

Key Point: *Always ask yourself: Is the regimen we are using meeting our needs? If not, change the plan. Don't settle.*

Plan Your Treatment Approach for Each Season: "Preventive" vs. "As-Needed" Medications

While you may think the "as needed" approach will result in less medication, sometimes the reverse is true. Several years ago I realized that if I take a combination of daily medications from early to mid-April to July 4, I felt better and actually took less medication than when I waited until I really needed it.

With the as-needed approach, my symptoms snowballed. By mid-May I was gulping over-the-counter pills and trying every nasal spray and eye remedy I could find.

With children, each year can be different. Your doctor should be able to guide you, and the best strategy is to continually revisit this question: "Should I keep my child on daily preventive medicine for the next couple of months or not?"

Decide on Oral vs. Topical Medications, or Both

Allergy specialists don't always agree on whether it is better to start with oral medications such as antihistamines or topical medications such as nose sprays. Theoretically, it is nice to stick to topical medications to avoid systemic side effects. But young kids often hate nose sprays, particularly the watery kinds that drip down the back of the throat. If your child also suffers from asthma, itchy eyes, or rashes, she may benefit from the systemic effects of an oral antihistamine. Oral medications make the most sense for occasional use. Most of the preferred nose sprays take a few days to work and are best used preventively. Find what works best for your child.

Consider Allergy Shots (Immunotherapy)

Sometimes hay fever symptoms are inadequately controlled with medications, and allergy shots should be considered (see Chapter 7). Allergy shots can help, but only you can decide whether it is worth it. Remember, since it often takes six months to a year to see significant improvement, your child is still going to require medications.

Key Point: *A good allergist will first explore other options before recommending allergy shots for a child with hay fever.*

Be Alert to the Complications of Hay Fever

Since children rarely complain of headaches or the other classic symptoms of sinus infections, pediatricians did not always appreciate that young children can develop sinusitis. Now we know sinus infections—whether bacterial, viral, and even fungal—can complicate inadequately controlled hay fever. If your child is not doing well, ask your healthcare provider if a sinus infection may be playing a role.

Optimize Therapy by Continually Reevaluating the Medical Approach

Ask yourself regularly, "Am I happy with my child's hay fever control?" For anyone, allergen exposure fluctuates widely from day to day and even from morning to night, and therefore, you need to continually think about adjustment of the medication. Find a medical practitioner who is willing to take your phone calls and advise you on a regular basis. Parents sometimes feel that this form of allergies is relatively minor so they decide not to bother their pediatrician or allergist. Nonsense! If these symptoms are bothering your child, they are important.

Specific Medications for Allergic Rhinitis

ANTIHISTAMINES

Antihistamines are a mainstay of therapy for children with allergies. They have been available for more than fifty years, and many are inexpensive over-the-counter drugs. One of the ironies of this field is that sometimes the so-called first-generation antihistamines, such as Benadryl or diphenhydramine, will give stronger and more immediate relief than newer prescription antihistamines. But while they are effective, some of these over-the-counter first-generation medications may cause more side effects (usually sleepiness and dizziness) than prescription varieties, and their effectiveness often wears off more quickly than some of the newer medications. So rather than grab the first allergy medicine you find at the drugstore, you'd be wise to consult the doctor—she may agree that over-the-counter medications are just right, or you may decide your child will be better served by a prescription medicine that will be longer lasting.

First-generation antihistamines

There are a bewildering, constantly changing variety of antihistamine-containing products, but only a few actual first-generation antihistamines (listed below) contained within these products. The primary differences have to do with how the medication is taken (syrups, tablets, time-release preparations) and with what they may be combined.

There is almost no scientific data that honestly compare these medications, and that is because responses vary from child to child. If you have found a favorite for your youngster, that's very likely the best one to use. Color and taste are important, just ask your child. Keep in mind that recommended doses on the bottles or boxes are really just guidelines; your doctor may alter the dosage. A higher dose may work better, but the more you give, the more side effects you can expect. There's no free lunch.

Drowsiness is a common side effect; while this isn't a problem for medications given before bed, it's certainly a problem for children during the day. Paradoxically, a small percentage of children have the opposite reaction and actually become keyed-up from antihistamines. This seems to be particularly true in children who are already considered active. Parents who are concerned about their child's attention span should consider whether antihistamines may be playing a role.

First-generation agents combined with decongestants are very helpful in controlling nasal congestion associated with "colds" or respiratory infections.

My personal preference for the child who is having severe allergy symptoms is a good slug of a first-generation antihistamine like Benadryl. However, for daily use, the newer prescription antihistamines are safer and last longer.

FIRST-GENERATION VS. THIRD-GENERATION ANTIHISTAMINES

First-Generation	Third-Generation
• Usually don't require a prescription	• Most require a prescription
• Very fast acting, but usually wears off quickly	• Long duration of action makes these very convenient for regular use
• Often very effective in high enough doses	• Generally very well tolerated with minimal side effects
• In general, may have more side effects (sleepiness, dry mouth, headaches, etc.)	
• More helpful for respiratory infections, particularly combined with decongestants	

Third-generation antihistamines

The four biggies in this group are loratadine (Claritin), fexofenadine (Allegra), cetirizine (Zyrtec), and the newest, desloratadine (Clarinex). They are generally very well tolerated, though children may still get sleepy if the dose is increased. You notice I skipped the second-generation of antihistamines. These medications had unacceptable side effects and are no longer available in the United States.

These newer medications tend to last longer than first-generation antihistamines. Because they take an hour or two before realizing full effect, they are best used before exposure to an allergen. The child who wakes up sneezing (perhaps in reaction to dust mites) would do best to take their medication at night before bed. If your child's biggest problem occurs while playing baseball in the afternoon, then a morning dose makes sense.

Although these medications are advertised to last twenty-four hours, this may not always be the case. Children metabolize any medications more quickly and effectively than do adults. If you notice that the effectiveness subsides late in the day, discuss with your child's physician whether you should try a twelve-hour preparation.

For young children with hay fever, Zyrtec and Claritin are available as syrups, so these are the two that are most often prescribed. For school-age kids who don't want syrups but still can't quite swallow pills, Claritin also comes in a clever rapidly dissolving tablet that kids place on their tongue, called Claritin Reditab. As with the first-generation agents, third-generation antihistamines are difficult to compare fairly. Each child responds differently, so don't give up because the first medicine you tried didn't work. Experiment with a few to learn which one works best for your child.

One member of this drug class, azelastine (Astelin), is

available in the United States as a topical spray. Kids tend not to like daily nose sprays—most prefer pills or liquids. However, Astelin can be added to a regimen for children who have bad hay fever and for whom a combination of medications might work.

Loratidine (Claritin) is now available both in generic form and without prescription, and others in this group may follow suit. This is the least sedating of the group, but the allergy symptoms of many children may not be adequately controlled by loratadine alone. If you don't feel your child is well controlled, speak up. Ask your physician about trying one of the other third-generation antihistamines or about adding a second medication.

COMMON ANTIHISTAMINES

First-Generation (Over-the-Counter)		Third-Generation (Usually Prescription)	
Generic Name	Sample Brand Names	Generic Name	Brand Name
brompheniramine	Dimetapp	loratadine	Claritin
chlorpheniramine	Chlortrimeton	cetirizine	Zyrtec
triprolidine	Actifed	fexofenadine	Allegra
clemastine	Tavist	azelastine	Astelin
diphenhydramine	Benadryl	desloratadine	Clarinex
promethazine	Phenergan		
cyproheptadine	Periatin		
azatadine	Optimine		
hydroxyzine	Atarax, Vistaril		

I am often asked whether it is safe to use antihistamines when your child with hay fever also has asthma. There is a legitimate concern that they may make asthma worse, particularly older nonprescription antihistamines. To avoid this problem, make sure your child's asthma is under good control. Then antihistamines can be safely used; by blocking allergic reactions, they may even help with your child's asthma control.

Decongestants

Antihistamines alone are often effective for sneezing and itching, but sometimes it is necessary to add a decongestant to help with nasal congestion and postnasal drip. Side effects from decongestants (tremors, sleeplessness, overdrying) can be significant, and these medications should generally be avoided for infants less than one year of age.

The most common oral decongestant is pseudoephedrine, often called by the brand name Sudafed. This agent is the active ingredient in many products, both over-the-counter and prescription, alone or combined with other drugs in syrups, chewable tablets, or pills. It can be prepared as either short-acting or in a time-release form.

Sometimes congestion is best relieved with a decongestant nasal spray. They are very effective and rapidly reduce nasal secretions and congestion. The oldest is phenylephrine (such as Neosynephrine), which is short-acting. The newer longer-acting medications in this family include oxymetazoline (such as Afrin).

The problem with these nasal sprays is that they are almost too good. After more than just a few days of use, you might find that your child seems to need them for weeks or months, as they can eventually lead to swelling of the membranes (known as "rebound swelling"). Therefore, limit these to only a few days at a time, when nasal congestion is severe. These medications can also cause side effects including burning, sneezing, and over-drying of the nasal membranes.

Atrovent nasal spray, a topical decongestant relatively new to the United States, contains ipatroprium bromide, an agent commonly used as an inhaler by adults with chronic bronchitis and sometimes asthma. This medication is what is known as anti-cholinergic and works by a different mechanism than other decongestants. It comes in two different strengths, and its role in allergic rhinitis is still being determined.

Decongestants can be useful as "add-on" therapy when antihistamines or other medications are not adequate, but they should be used cautiously. If continued use is necessary, it should be carefully supervised by your physician.

CHROMONES

Cromolyn sodium nose sprays, such as Nasalcrom, are safe and effective in controlling allergic rhinitis, but they don't do much for respiratory infections. This medication no longer requires a prescription and while it's not as effective as nasal steroids, many kids respond very well. There is very little marketing going on for this medication, and many physicians don't think of using it, but the safety profile of this agent is very reassuring for parents and pediatricians. For cromolyn to be effective, your child must take it every day, often two or three times a day, and its benefits may not be seen for days or even weeks.

NASAL STEROIDS

Inhaled corticosteroids are currently the mainstay of asthma treatment, and likewise they are very important medications when used as a nasal spray for allergic rhinitis. This treatment works by directly suppressing the inflammation within the nose, markedly decreasing the sneezing, congestion, and itching of hay fever. These sprays may take from a couple of days to a couple of weeks to build up their effect, so they are best used as preventive therapy for your child's allergy season. More effective than cromolyn, they seem to control the nasal symptoms of allergies better than any other medications.

Children with bad allergies tend to have symptoms year-round, and many parents and pediatricians are reluctant to keep their children on nasal corticosteroids for long periods of time. There is a lot of misinformation out there about this family of medications (refer to Chapter 13). Remember that nasal sprays result in very small doses absorbed into the systemic circulation, and the risk of side effects is small.

One advantage of nasal steroid sprays is that you don't have to worry about any drug interactions or behavioral effects as you might with antihistamines or decongestants. But there are some downsides to nasal steroids. They are designed for daily preventive therapy and rarely work immediately so they are not the "drug of choice" for quick relief. These nasal sprays can cause local side effects, such as burning, sneezing, or even nosebleeds. In addition, young children tend to dislike nose sprays—an unwilling child can make the use of a nasal spray a real family battle, severely limiting their use.

The list of medications in this family continues to grow, and I can't hope to be up to date here. Current nasal steroid inhalers and sprays include beclomethasone (Beconase AQ and Vancenase AQ), triamcinolone (Nasacort), fluticasone (Flonase), budesonide (Rhinocort AQ), flunisolide (Nasarel and Nasalide), and mometasone (Nasonex). These are very effective and therefore represent a huge market. As a sufferer of chronic hay fever myself, I can tell you that the differences between products are not very great. Some children do seem to derive more benefit or have fewer side effects from one brand versus another. It really is a matter of trial and error.

Dry vs. aqueous

Nasal steroids were previously available in two forms: metered-dose inhalers and aqueous solutions. The metered-dose inhalers (MDI) were better tolerated by young children than the watery sprays, particularly if the aqueous sprays drip down the back of their nose into their mouth. But the MDIs are no longer available as they were propelled by CFCs, which are bad for the environment. For this reason, pharmaceutical companies currently only market the watery (aqueous) sprays. As a pediatrician, I am troubled by the lack of nasal sprays using safe propellants (known as HFA), since my young patients will not have access to this important option. I guess young children do not represent a large enough market for companies to develop an environmentally safe metered-dose nasal steroid inhaler.

Combining Medications

For children with bad hay fever, it is often better to combine medications. If your child only requires occasional medication for hay fever, this will usually mean starting with an oral antihistamine, with decongestants added for brief periods of time and nasal steroids added for longer seasons. The trick is consistency. If you start this preventive therapy even before your child's symptoms appear, you will likely be pleased with the result. If your child's nasal symptoms are worsening as the season continues, add a second medication. If your child is not adequately controlled with both oral antihistamines and nasal sprays, add decongestants or other medications.

While hay fever is not life-threatening, it can significantly impair your child's lifestyle. Whether it's feeling stuffed up all the time or sneezing through science class, there's nothing fun about itching, stuffiness, sneezing, and coughing with hay fever.

Somewhere out there is almost always a combination of medications that can safely and effectively control your child's symptoms without side effects. To optimize this strategy, have clear goals and continuously adjust medications to meet your child's needs. Call your doctor as often as needed until you feel that you've got this season's symptoms controlled. Then you may have to start again next season.

ALLERGIC CONJUNCTIVITIS

Many kids who suffer from allergic rhinitis also suffer with red and itchy eyes from allergic conjunctivitis. Your child's eyes may react to a variety of allergens or just to one or two. Some kids only have red itchy eyes when they are exposed to cats. Many are bothered during certain pollen seasons, such as tree or grass season. Others are bothered all year round. I think many physicians tend to focus on the nose and forget that itchy eyes are very uncomfortable. Kids hate this and so do I. Now these symptoms can be controlled.

Symptoms of Allergic Conjunctivitis

Both eyes are usually affected, though one may be worse than the other. The symptoms of allergic conjunctivitis usually include one or more of the following:

- Red, swollen conjunctivae
- Itching, burning, stinging
- Tearing or increased watery secretions
- Swollen eyelids

Key point: *There are many reasons for red eyes.*
If simple allergy medications don't
solve the problem, seek medical
attention.

Over time the diagnosis of allergic conjunctivitis usually is obvious. But remember that just like your skin, there are non-allergic triggers for red eyes, such as cosmetics or pollution. Also, kids can't resist rubbing eyes that are itchy, and they may become infected. If you see any pus, or if you are not certain, see a doctor.

Prevention of Allergic Conjunctivitis

In previous chapters I have already reviewed some of the ways you can try to minimize your child's exposure to allergens. Prevention is always preferable in theory but our goal is also to allow your child to live as normal a lifestyle as possible. So medications are often an important part of the therapy.

Management of allergic conjunctivitis

- Cold compresses give significant quick relief. In fact, here's a little trick: Keep any eye medications in the refrigerator, and your child will get relief as soon as the cooled solutions are instilled.

- Sometimes all that is needed are lubrication drops, such as "artificial tears" or other over-the-counter eye drops.

- Avoid the use of contact lenses during allergy season, especially those that remain in for a long period of times. These will just make everything worse.

- Over-the-counter decongestant eye drops help decrease redness but rarely help the itchiness that is the worst part of eye allergies. In fact, by drying the eyes, sometimes these medications can make things worse. So if you want to try these, pick up one that also contains a lubricant. And don't use it for more than a few days at a time.

- Over-the-counter antihistamine eye drops help a little, but I have been much more impressed with prescription versions.

- Since most children with bad eye allergies also have significant nasal symptoms, many will already be taking oral antihistamines. In my own experience, the dose required to help intense eye itching is quite high and leads to significant drowsiness. So adding a topical eye drop is often the way to go. There are a few different families of eye drops which I will briefly summarize below.

- Prescription eye drops can really help, but a bit of trial-and-error may be required. As with all medications, don't settle until you find one your child likes.

Key point: *As in all allergic reactions, the most effective medications are corticosteroid eye drops. However, there are very significant risks, and they usually should only be used as a last resort under the watchful eye of an eye doctor.*

CURRENTLY AVAILABLE NONSTEROIDAL PRESCRIPTION EYE DROPS FOR ALLERGIC CONJUNCTIVITIS

- Antihistamines:
    Emadine, Livostin, Optivar

- Mast cell stabilizers:
    Alocril, Alomet, Alomide, Crolom, Opticrom

- Combined antihistamine and mast cell stabilizers:
    Patanol, Zaditor

- NSAIDs (nonsteroidal anti-inflammatory drugs):
    Acular, Voltaren

TAKE-HOME MESSAGES

- Hay fever can be safely and effectively controlled by identifying the offending allergens and trying to minimize your child's contact with them.

- Treatment plans need to be considered seasonally and medications given either preventively or as needed.

- Immunotherapy can help hay fever, but most parents will prefer to first try to control their children's symptoms with medications.

- Hay fever can lead to complications, such as bacterial or fungal infections that require separate treatment. So be observant about your child's medical condition.

- Red and itchy eyes can be very annoying.
  Prescription eye drops designed for allergic
  conjunctivitis really help.

- Continually reevaluate how things are going.
  Your child's allergies may change over time,
  and new medications are constantly coming
  to the market.

- Chronic nasal congestion and sinus infections
  are not always caused by allergies. If allergy medications don't help, ask if your child could have
  another problem such as IgA deficiency or gastroesophageal reflux (see chapter 5).

EIGHTEEN

Skin Allergies

Skin is one of the most amazing parts of our bodies. The older my skin gets, the more I am impressed by the beautiful, smooth, blemish-free skin of infants and young children. The characteristic I admire most is skin's ability to heal itself despite almost constant injury and exposure to our environment. It is truly a miracle of nature.

Some people, though, have extremely sensitive skin that can be the source of relentless discomfort. If your child suffers from skin allergies, you are only too aware of the suffering that can occur. Eczema, hives, and other types of itchy or scaly skin rashes are often due to allergic reactions triggered by all sorts of things ranging from exposure to plants, chemicals, metals, or even food. Therapy for skin allergies continues to improve, and your child's symptoms can almost always be successfully controlled.

While it is tempting to reach for an over-the-counter ointment, a better plan is to work with your child's physicians and pin down the actual cause of the allergy. Avoidance is always the best policy, but when not practical, your doctor can prescribe a combination of allergy medications, ointments, or creams—or even antibiotics.

As with any type of allergy, the ideal solution is to prevent exposure. Sometimes identifying the cause of a skin problem is easy. If your daughter's earlobes become red and inflamed every time she wears a certain pair of earrings, get rid of those earrings. She is probably having an allergic reaction to nickel, a substance often present in inexpensive jewelry. Other times, making a diagnosis is more difficult. The trigger for recurrent hives is often elusive, and an experienced expert in allergies can really help.

Like all allergies, skin allergies come and go and may develop gradually over time in reaction to things that previously caused no difficulty. Consider food allergies. I remember a boy named Allen who loved peanut butter and jelly and ate it every day. His mother gradually noticed that he sometimes came home from school scratching his arms and legs. His hives would come and go and sometimes disappear for weeks.

Allen's mom spoke to his pediatrician and neither of them could figure out the trigger. They considered the peanut butter he loved so much but discounted that idea because he ate it every day and some weeks had no hives at all. It took at least two months before his mother figured it out. He only had hives when she bought one particular brand of strawberry jam for his sandwiches. To complicate matters, Allen could eat strawberries alone without any problem. The hives were related not to the strawberries but to the artificial coloring in that particular brand.

Goals for Management of Skin Allergies

Just as with hay fever or asthma, "no symptoms" needn't always be the goal. It may be okay to have a little eczema or an occasional itch. However, a child shouldn't feel itchy all of the time to the point of waking at night, and you don't want her scratching so much her skin becomes infected. You certainly don't want a child to be teased or embarrassed.

As usual, you want to give your child the least amount of medicine possible to control symptoms adequately. Even topical creams and lotions should be used with caution. Here are some basic steps to take with any chronic skin condition:

MOISTURIZE

If skin is dry, it becomes itchy and more sensitive to all kinds of irritants. So if dry is bad, does that mean water is good? No, too much water is a major cause of overly dry skin. Kids love to play in water, relax in the bathtub, and stay in the swimming pool for hours on end, but exposure to water leads to overdrying. If your child has a skin condition, your physician will advise you to keep soaking to a minimum.

Too much sun and wind are also very drying. Avoid detergents. Most bubble baths are a real no-no. Bland cleansing agents or moisturizing soaps with a neutral pH (nonacidic) such as Dove can be used in moderation. Avoid preparations that have perfumes or preservatives. And when your children finally do climb out of the bath or pool, pat them dry with a towel, don't rub vigorously. Apply a moisturizer when the skin is still moist. (Ointments or creams tend to be more effective than lotions.)

PREVENT SCRATCHING

Itching triggers scratching, which triggers more itching, and that vicious cycle leads to skin infections, which can lead to chronic skin problems. It is very difficult to stop your child from scratching when her skin is dry and itchy. That's why your first goal is to moisturize the skin to try to prevent it from being dry and itchy. Then keep your child's nails short and clean, though this is easier said than done.

SPECIFIC SKIN CONDITIONS

Here are some common conditions that can occur:

Atopic dermatitis (eczema)

Eczema is a general term for inflamed skin and can appear anywhere on the body. There are many reasons for skin to be inflamed, but we will focus on a common type of eczema, atopic dermatitis, which presents as patches of dry, itchy inflamed skin most often affecting the insides of the elbows, in back of the knees, and on the face. Because these patches are intensely itchy, it is almost impossible to stop scratching. Scratching then leads to weeping or crusted sores that may become infected. Along with hay fever and asthma, chronic eczema is included in the category of atopic diseases because children who are chronically affected almost always have other types of allergies. Many infants have eczema that resolves over the first few years of life, but in some children these rashes continue to appear off and on throughout their childhood. When eczema flares up it is not only very itchy and painful, it can be very embarrassing.

What triggers atopic dermatitis? The immediate trigger is not always obvious. Sometimes heat or sweating seems to be a cause. Exercise probably doesn't trigger flares on its own, but by triggering sweating, eczema often worsens. Low humidity causes drying of the skin, again leading to itching and flaking and the vicious cycle of scratch and itch. Soaps, detergents, perfumes, allergens, infections, and even stress can also contribute to a reaction. Children with atopic dermatitis have such sensitive skin that they often develop flushing and itching when they are upset or angry, which easily progresses into full-blown eczema.

Skin testing for allergens may be difficult in kids with

atopic dermatitis. Their skin is often so sensitive that just the act of scratching can trigger a significant hive or area of inflammation, making false-positive skin tests common.

Management of atopic dermatitis. Prevention is clearly the best approach, but kids with atopic dermatitis will have occasional flare-ups. With young children, parents are more likely to catch eczema in the early stage and symptoms can be minimized. As they grow older, parents often miss the first few days of a rash, when it is still possible to intervene. Teach your kids that it is to their benefit to let you know if their skin is starting to itch or redden. Then you can make sure that everything is being done to control itching and minimize scratching.

Patches of eczema are prone to infection. If you and your child learn how to recognize early signs of infection, such as increased redness, fluid-filled blisters (pustules), or even cold sores or fever blisters, then appropriate antibiotics or antiviral medications can be started right away. Ultraviolet light or sunlamps, sometimes used for severe eczema, should only be done under the careful guidance of a dermatologist.

Allergy shots may help hay fever and possibly asthma, but they rarely have proven effective for atopic dermatitis. Many nutritional approaches have been suggested, but I am not aware of any scientific evidence to support their use.

Suggested Strategies for Atopic Dermatitis

- Establish a realistic daily skin care regimen.
- Help your child to recognize stress in their life and how to deal with it.
- Work to minimize scratching.
- Avoid allergens and irritants.
- Watch for infection.
- Moisturize, moisturize, moisturize.

Contact dermatitis (nonallergic)

Burning, stinging, itching, and redness of the skin, may not be allergic, it may just be an irritation. Common skin irritants include bath soaps, detergents, cosmetics, antiperspirants, moisturizers, and all kinds of hair care products. Irritated dry skin just from water is probably the most common skin problem of all.

Contact dermatitis (allergic)

Some chemicals trigger allergic reactions. Nickel in jewelry is a good example, and fragrances and the preservatives in many cosmetics and skin products can cause full-blown allergic reactions. Your daughter may not react immediately to a new makeup or perfume because sometimes it takes a few days of repeated use for symptoms to appear. To further confuse the situation, many reactions take an hour or more to occur, and some reactions to fragrances don't occur until the skin is exposed to sunlight. Some cosmetics and fragrances are promoted as "hypoallergenic." This does not mean "can't cause allergies," only that the product is less likely to cause allergic reactions.

If you've found your child reacts to fragrances, pay attention to labeling. Some fragrances are added to products to mask other chemical odors, so "unscented" doesn't mean "fragrance-free." If you want items that have absolutely nothing added for scent reasons, then the product should be marked "fragrance-free" or "without perfume."

Preservatives are added to many products and are important in preventing them from going bad. Some common preservatives are DMDM hydantoin, formaldehyde, imidazolidinyl urea, methylchloroisothiazolinone, paraben, phenoxyethanol, and Quaternium-15. If your child seems to be having an allergic reaction to a particular product, write down all of the ingredients. Many children can tolerate some preservatives but not others. Over time you'll be able to identify which ones are causing the problems.

Hives (urticaria and angioedema)

Hives, or urticaria, are red bumps or patches on the skin that appear suddenly. When the skin is even slightly irritated, a red swelling can develop and trigger itching.

Determining the cause of hives can be difficult. My wife had been suffering on and off for weeks, and I'd asked her all my usual allergy questions: "Have you changed your laundry detergent? Are you wearing any new clothing? When else have you suffered from hives?" Finally we identified the culprit— fabric softener dryer sheets. It took us a while to figure this out because she didn't develop hives every time she wore newly washed and dried clothing. That was because the fabric softener wasn't evenly distributed on the clothing, and only some pieces were sufficiently coated to trigger hives.

Hives may result from other causes including allergies to medications, usually occurring within an hour of ingestion. To complicate matters, hives may not be caused by the active ingredients but rather by the preservatives, flavorings, colorings, stabilizing agents, and other ingredients in modern medications. Hives can, of course, also be due to food allergies (fully described in Chapter 11).

Sometimes the location of the hives provides a clue as to the cause. For instance, if a child has an allergic reaction to something he ate or to a drug, hives may appear all over, but if he has a reaction to direct irritation from a piece of clothing or rubber, he might have hives only at the point where the skin comes in contact with the offending item. Acute hives are usually gone in just a few hours, but sometimes last for weeks.

The following measures will provide some relief:

- Gently apply cool or lukewarm cloths or compresses.
- Avoid tight-fitting clothes over the affected area.
- Don't use hot water or strong soaps or detergents.
- Medications, particularly antihistamines, may help control itching and will eventually help bring the swelling down.

Angioedema: Hive Look-Alikes That Can Trigger an Emergency

Skin allergies can cause swelling beneath the skin instead of just on the surface. This kind of deep swelling (angioedema) can be very serious, and it usually lasts longer than regular hives. If angioedema occurs on the tongue or throat the windpipe can swell and narrow, causing difficulty breathing and creating a medical emergency. If hives or swelling occur with any of the following symptoms, contact a doctor immediately:

- Difficulty breathing
- Chest pain or "tightness"
- Wheezing
- Swelling of the lips, tongue, or face

If swelling spreads over large areas or your child is having any of the above symptoms, don't rely on antihistamines. Get immediate medical attention for either an injection of epinephrine (adrenaline) or steroids or both.

Latex allergy

Latex or natural rubber is the milky sap from rubber trees, and clever inventors have found thousands of ways to utilize this naturally occurring chemical. As the number of uses for latex has grown, so has the number or reports of allergic reactions.

The most common reactions are skin-related, but some people have had much more severe responses from inhaling small particles of latex in powder form. Nurses and physicians who wear latex gloves are the highest risk group, but patients exposed to latex during various medical, surgical, and dental procedures have also developed latex allergy.

EXAMPLES OF MEDICAL PRODUCTS
THAT OFTEN CONTAIN LATEX

Gloves	Stethoscopes
Blood pressure cuffs	Rubber stoppers for vials and syringes
EKG electrodes	Intravenous tubing
Dental dams	Tourniquets

Latex is also found in many products in the home, including pacifiers, nipples for baby bottles, rubber toys, adhesives, elastic in clothing, shower curtains, carpeting, and of course, balloons.

More than half of kids born with spina bifida develop a latex allergy, so it is important that parents of these children routinely avoid latex. This is very important since these children often require many medical or surgical procedures, during which exposure to latex is quite common.

Symptoms of latex allergy. The symptoms of latex allergy

can be subtle or severe. They include all of the usual symptoms of an allergic reaction including itching, red skin, hives, and swelling (angioedema). If the respiratory system is exposed your child may develop signs of allergic rhinitis (sneezing, runny or congested nose), scratchy throat, hoarseness, cough, or even wheezing. Rarely, latex allergy can trigger full-blown anaphylactic shock with flushing, vomiting, cramps, difficulty breathing, swelling of the tongue and throat, or a sudden drop of blood pressure that leads to loss of consciousness.

Many people who are allergic to latex are naturally worried about plants that may secrete latexlike chemicals such as poinsettia and rubber plants. These chemicals can potentially cause allergic reactions, but they are rarely a problem, probably because the exposure is usually low. However, if your child is highly allergic to latex, it is probably prudent to be wary of these and other latex-containing plants.

The proteins in some foods are similar to those in latex, so kids who are allergic to latex may also become allergic to chestnuts, avocado, and bananas. There are many other foods (potato, kiwi, cantaloupe, and tomato) that may also have proteins similar to latex, though the evidence of so-called cross-reactivity with latex is less.

Latex paint is not a problem, since these paints do not contain natural rubber or latex. Rather they contain synthetics that are not really related to the naturally occurring proteins that can trigger these reactions. Don't worry about shiny newspaper pages—they are coated with synthetics, not natural rubber or latex.

Preventing latex exposure. If your child is allergic to latex, you need to get in the habit of reading product labels very carefully. If it is unclear, contact the manufacturer and ask.

In the United States, all medical devices and their packaging have been required to be labeled as to latex content since 1998. However, some pharmaceutical products and medications are still stored in bottles that have rubber stoppers. I particularly worry about medication vials, since the rubber stopper may be punctured repeatedly with needles to withdraw liquid medications. All of us need to encourage the pharmaceutical industry to replace all rubber stoppers with synthetic products.

Stick to balloons that don't contain natural rubber, such as those made of Mylar. As your child gets older, it will be important to tell him that there are alternatives to latex condoms.

If your child has spina bifida or latex allergy and requires a surgical procedure, make sure that it is performed in surgical suites that are specifically designed to be latex-free. Most hospitals are well aware of this problem and should have a complete latex-free protocol developed, including staff education about latex allergy.

Testing for latex allergy. Skin testing and blood testing for latex allergy can be done, but there are many false negatives. Latex contains many different proteins that can trigger allergic reactions, so completely accurate testing is not yet possible.

Treatment for latex allergy. All of the same types of treatment used for other allergic reactions are useful for latex allergy. Skin reactions can be treated with steroid creams and antihistamines to control itching. Asthma medications are useful if latex triggers coughing or wheezing. And, of course, epinephrine (adrenaline) is essential if a severe or anaphylactic reaction occurs. I do not know of any forms of therapy, such as allergy shots, used to desensitize someone with latex allergy, so recognition of the problem is important.

Given the potential severity of these reactions, if your child is known to be allergic to latex, it is important that they wear a Medic-Alert bracelet or necklace.

"Leaves of Three, Let Them Be"

Poison ivy is most often found in the eastern and central regions of the United States, though it can grow almost anywhere. Poison oak is most common in the west. It looks similar to poison ivy, though the underside of the leaves have a lighter green color and are covered with "hair." Poison oak sometimes has berries. Just to really confuse you, one variety of poison ivy, usually found in the southeast, looks more like poison oak and is even called "eastern poison oak." Incidentally, neither poison ivy nor poison oak will grow above an elevation of about 4,000 feet.

Poison ivy may grow as low shrubs or as vines, and it sometimes has yellow-green flowers and greenish white berries. Look out for plants with groups of three glossy green leaves. As the saying goes, "Leaves of three, let them be."

Poison sumac is a tree that usually stands about five or six feet high. If your kids like to hike in the woods— particularly in swampy areas—this is a plant to watch for. Like poison oak, poison sumac trees often have clusters of green berries drooping below the branches. (Non-poisonous sumac trees have red berries.)

Poison Ivy, Poison Oak, and Poison Sumac

Captain John Smith wrote about this common form of skin allergy soon after arriving in North America, and some experts have estimated that almost 85 percent of us will develop an allergic reaction to poison ivy, oak, or sumac in our lifetimes. Like any allergic reaction, there is no sensitivity if there has been no prior exposure. Even after a child's sensitivity has been established, the allergic reaction is not immediate. The intense itching and rash usually don't occur until twelve to forty-eight hours after exposure (though the delay can vary from four hours to a few days). In the classic reaction, the skin turns red and blisters, bumps, itching, and sometimes swelling generally follow. Eventually those blisters will break and ooze before crusting over and fading away. Usually the reaction worsens over time, peaking in about five days and resolving within about two weeks, even with no treatment. The most common complication is bacterial infection of the skin sores, usually introduced by scratching. Very rarely, the allergic reaction spreads over the body and can trigger serious overall illness.

Very severe reactions can occur when someone makes the mistake of using poison sumac branches for firewood. The chemical is in the smoke from burning plants, and in susceptible people inhaling the smoke can cause allergic reactions in the nose and respiratory tract, as well as on the skin.

The stuff that causes the reaction, urushiol, can remain active for a year or longer. So it is important to wash any plant resin off clothing, garden tools, and fishing or hunting gear with soap and water. Children can develop poison ivy rash just by coming in contact with this resin left on someone else's clothing. While most kids develop reactions when playing outdoors during the warm weather, poison ivy can occur in the winter, since the resin that triggers the reaction is still present in dead or decaying plants.

Since the chemical is not in the fluid that oozes from the blister, the rash is not spread by scratching or bathing. For the same reason, you don't have to worry about either you or your child developing a rash by touching someone else's rash.

By the way, dogs and cats usually don't react to these plants, but the resin on their fur can definitely rub off on you later. So unless your family pet is wearing gloves, shirts, and pants, remember to bathe them thoroughly if you think they may have been exposed.

Teach your children how to identify poison ivy, oak, and sumac so they can avoid contact as much as possible (see sidebar on page 328). In addition, encourage your children to wear gloves, long sleeves, and long pants when they are tramping around in the woods. (After you have done that, make sure to get them to do all of their homework before watching TV and put their dishes in the sink.) Actually, it's amazing that every kid isn't covered by poison ivy rashes all of the time.

Key Point: *Don't assume your children are not susceptible to poison ivy, oak, or sumac even if they have been exposed multiple times. The next time could be the one that triggers an allergic reaction.*

Treatment of poison ivy, poison oak, or poison sumac. The sores from poison ivy, poison oak, and poison sumac will heal on their own, but cold compresses can help relieve itching and irritation when the rash is oozing. These compresses can be soaked in plain water or a diluted solution of liquid aluminum acetate known as "Burrow's solution." Calamine lotion helps to dry the rash and relieve itching. Some parents find that soaking in a lukewarm oatmeal bath, sometimes with a little baking soda added, can be very soothing.

There are many over-the-counter and prescription preparations designed for poison ivy, but use these conservatively. When skin is already inflamed, many of these products, like sprays of mild anesthetics like lidocaine or benzocaine, can themselves trigger a chemical skin reaction.

A promising new product, bentoquatam (IvyBlock), has recently been introduced. By spraying this over-the-counter lotion on skin at least fifteen minutes before exposure to poison ivy, oak, or sumac, a reaction can sometimes be prevented or at least the severity of any rash can be significantly decreased. If your child is sensitive to poison ivy, reapply bentoquatam approximately every four hours to maintain protection. This product is not yet recommended for children age six or younger. If your child's rash seems to worsen after using these compounds, stop them immediately.

If the rash covers large areas of your child's body or if it is on their face or genitals, call the doctor. Antihistamines, topical and oral steroids, can help control the itching and inflammation, but even topical creams and lotions need to be used cautiously.

General Treatments for Skin Irritations

Sometimes the best treatment is systemic, other times you want to treat topically. Here are some of the possibilities for managing a skin condition:

Antihistamines

(Also refer to Chapter 17 for more information on antihistamines.)

When antihistamines are prescribed for use with skin allergies, the goal is to control itching. Some of the older antihistamines (first-generation medicines) work very well, so many allergists and dermatologists will recommend hydroxyzine (Atarax or Vistaril) or diphenhydramine (Benadryl). However, these older medications usually wear off quickly and can be sedating. For daily use, the newer antihistamines—Allegra, Claritin, Clarinex, and Zyrtec—are preferred.

While antihistamines are reasonably effective, every child responds differently. If your child is not improving—or if he is groggy from the antihistamine—consult your doctor. There will be something else to try.

TOPICAL STEROIDS

The judicious use of steroid creams, lotions, and ointments is the main form of treatment for severe itching and redness of skin allergies. There are literally dozens of choices, so work closely with your physician to find the ones that help your child.

Hydrocortisone, which now comes in diluted over-the-counter concentrations, is quite safe, but often inadequate. The more potent steroids can lead to thinning of the skin and permanent red marks known to physicians as either *telangiectasia,* which are fine red lines, often "spidery" looking, or *striae,* which are larger, longer red marks, usually in skin creases. One type of steroid product known as *fluorinated glucocorticosteroids* are known to leave red marks on skin and are usually not prescribed for use on the face.

While the stronger steroid creams can be highly effective, they also may have significant long-term risks. Chronic heavy use of topical steroids can result in some absorption of the steroids and the long-term side effects of oral prednisone, such as slow growth, high blood pressure, and muscle weakness. Use the mildest steroid agents that work for the shortest period possible.

ANTIBIOTICS OR ANTISEPTICS

Skin irritations can become infected, especially if children scratch a lot. Many creams and lotions are now available with antiseptics or antibiotics in them, sometimes combined with steroids. Oral antibiotics may be needed for severely infected skin.

IMMUNE-MODULATING AGENTS

Until recently steroid preparations were really the only choice for treatment of atopic dermatitis, but now there is a new family of medications receiving FDA approval. The first two medicines, tacrolimis (Protopic) and pimecrolimus (Elidel), appear to be safer than chronically used steroids, and other members of this class should soon be available. The dermatologists or allergists to whom I make my referrals for skin conditions are reporting back great results with these new agents.

OTHER PREPARATIONS

Your physician might use other preparations in specific situations. For instance, if your child happens to have skin patches that are oozing or weeping, then drying agents might be temporarily required. Very thickened dry skin may require *keratolytics* that help break down the thickened skin so new skin can grow.

TAKE-HOME MESSAGES

- Keeping your child's skin from being too dry is the first step toward preventing skin problems. Use moisturizers, and keep nails short to reduce scratching.

- Rather than treating a chronic problem with over-the-counter medications, check with your doctor and get a diagnosis. This will broaden your treatment options, and you may find something that works more effectively.

- Work with your doctor to try and pinpoint the causes of allergic skin reactions. Once you know the cause, it will be easier to help your child avoid the problem.

- Some skin conditions can become infected. If you notice increased redness, blisters, pustules, or even cold sores or fever blisters, check with your doctor about getting antibiotics or antiviral medications.

- Teach your child to avoid classic triggers such as poison ivy and poison oak.

- Children with latex allergy can have quite severe reactions. If you think your child is allergic to latex, talk to your doctor and begin practicing latex avoidance.

NINETEEN

Drug and Insect Allergies

Anyone who has had a serious reaction to a medication or an insect sting quickly learns to respect these allergies. Unfortunately, children with allergies aren't born with labels. You can only discover your child is allergic to bees after his first, second, or third insect sting. (Remember, allergies develop over time and exposure to the allergen.) The same holds true with drug allergies. You may have treated your child's ear infections numerous times with a specific antibiotic, and then one night hives develop . . . leaving you to wonder if it's the drug.

If your child has a reaction to either insect stings or medications, it's important to identify whether he is allergic or intolerant. True allergic reactions to these stimuli can be life-threatening, so once an allergy has been identified you will want to teach your child to practice avoidance and what to do in case of an unexpected reaction.

Allergies to Medicines

The older I get, the more conservative I've become when it comes to prescribing drugs for children. Why use up any medications we have for fighting serious infections if the illness doesn't really merit it?

Children have a wonderful ability to digest and metabolize

just about anything prescribed for them, and they tolerate medications much better than adults. And while those incredibly long lists of potential side effects in the package inserts are more likely to apply to adults than kids, every pediatrician can tell you of patients who develop significant allergic reactions and side effects from medications that have been safely tolerated by hundreds of children over the years. Suffice it to say, the fewer drugs to which your child is exposed, the less likely he or she is to develop an allergy.

Key Point: *There is no free lunch. Any*
medication that actually helps
a child must also potentially
cause side effects. I'm afraid
this is a law of nature.

Allergic reactions to a prescribed drug may occur on the first dose or may build over time, catching parents by surprise. Did a virus cause the rash? Are hives part of the disease? What about the new acne cream or an antibiotic? As with any allergy, careful observation and some detective work are almost always necessary. You may need to consult a specialist. Drug allergies are potentially so serious that it's vital your child not be exposed again to that drug or related medications.

As you know by now, an allergic reaction is triggered by the body's immune system, starting with production of this molecule, IgE, and leading to a cascade of chemical reactions that result in itching, hives, sneezing, coughing, and swelling. The most common form of drug hypersensitivity generally produces a skin rash (hives) but can affect any organ in the body. Fevers, joint pains, coughing, wheezing, and rarely generalized anaphylaxis can occur. Allergic reactions may sometimes damage the heart, lungs, and kidneys. I have seen really nasty generalized allergic reactions, some of which have resulted in prolonged stays in our pediatric intensive care unit. In my experience, most children who have very serious reactions continued to take the medication involved long after side effects had begun. Pay attention to any curious symptoms that develop when your child is taking any type of medication—even if she has been on it before.

Key Point: **If you think your child may be developing an allergic reaction, stop giving the medication immediately and speak to your doctor. Don't take a chance.**

If you and your doctor aren't certain whether your child has had an allergic reaction, see an allergist. Both skin testing and blood tests for drug allergies can be done, but they are tricky to interpret. This should be done by an expert.

Though our focus is on allergies, there are many types of adverse reactions to drugs and sometimes the problem is caused by interactions between drugs. Tell all your children's doctors about any other medications she may be taking.

Missed Cues

Parents often discount the possibility of a drug reaction because their child tolerated that same medication so many times before. Because allergic reactions develop only after repeated exposure, don't be shocked if your child develops a reaction from something she tolerated before. And while drug reactions, like other allergic reactions, most often occur within an hour or less of exposure, there may be a delay since it takes time for a medication to be absorbed into the system.

While most drug rashes fade quickly after medication is stopped (more than a few hours), allergic rashes can actually come and go for days or weeks afterward. Many medications are first broken down into smaller chemicals before they are excreted. These breakdown products, or drug metabolites, may continue to trigger allergic reactions if they contain part of the chemical structure that triggered the reaction in the first place.

A Rash Doesn't Always Mean Allergy

The most common example of a drug reaction mistakenly thought to be allergic is a fine rash that occurs in about 5 to 10 percent of kids taking amoxicillin or ampicillin. Amoxicillin is the antibiotic most commonly prescribed by pediatricians in the United States. If your child develops a fine red rash— either flat or slightly raised, often all over the trunk and extremities—she may have the typical rash that sometimes occurs with amoxicillin. This rash is not dangerous and usually occurs when a child has a virus. Many parents mistakenly believe their child is now allergic to amoxicillin. Check with your doctor to get a definitive diagnosis.

Key Point: *The benign rash of amoxicillin is not itchy, and allergic rashes usually are. Report your observation to the doctor as it will help her make a diagnosis.*

Reactions Aren't Always to the Drug Itself

Ingredients are often added to liquid medicines as preservatives or to make them taste better, but these extra ingredients sometimes trigger reactions. Sometimes a child can safely be given the pill form of the medicine though she had a reaction to the liquid.

Ironically, even asthma inhalers may contain ingredients that can trigger allergic reactions. For instance, some inhalers contain soy lecithin, which is a distant cousin to nuts. And the new dry powder inhalers contain lactose, which is derived from milk and potentially could be contaminated with tiny amounts of milk protein.

PSEUDOALLERGIC REACTIONS CAN ALSO BE THREATENING

Some nonallergic reactions mimic true allergic reactions and can be very confusing—as well as quite serious. Pseudoallergic reactions are fairly common, and an allergist can be quite helpful in pinpointing what is going on. Reactions to contrast material used in so many fancy X-ray tests are examples of allergiclike reactions. While this reaction is not actually a true IgE-mediated allergic reaction, it can be very serious. Someone who has a reaction to these dyes may react again each time they are exposed. Unlike a true allergic reaction, the severity of the reaction doesn't necessarily increase with repeated exposure.

THE IMPORTANCE OF IDENTIFICATION

If your child has had a true allergic reaction, with rare exceptions, they should never again be given that drug or chemically similar drugs. The next time they are exposed, the reaction could be worse. On the other hand, if the reaction was not allergic, then there is no reason to avoid that medication, which may be safer than the alternatives. That's why it is important to consult your doctor for a definite answer.

Severe Drug Reactions

For an anaphylactic reaction, see Chapter 20. Keep these points in mind:

- Symptoms of drug reactions (itching, hives, sneezing, wheezing, coughing, swelling, etc.) may come and go, often for more than twenty-four hours and sometimes for weeks.
- Obtain a medic-alert bracelet or necklace that names any medications to which your child is allergic, and make sure they always wear it.
- Keep handy an anaphylactic kit with epinephrine (adrenaline) in the appropriate strength for your child. Know how and when to use it, and make sure your epinephrine has not expired.

Key Point: *If your child is having trouble breathing or is describing a tight feeling in his mouth, throat, or chest, dial 911 or 0 (operator).*

Management of a Possible Drug Allergy

- Don't give your child any more of a medication if you suspect an allergy.
- Call 911 or the operator if your child is having trouble breathing or is experiencing swelling in the mouth or throat.
- Call your child's doctor to discuss what has happened.

- Don't count on anyone else, including physicians or pharmacists, to remember your child's drug allergies. Any time your child is prescribed a new medication, ask if it is related. Check with your pharmacist about any over-the-counter medications.
- If you and your child's doctor decide to try a medication that may have caused a reaction in the past, give it in your doctor's office the first time and plan to stay there for at least forty minutes to watch for reactions.
- The itching of hives or other rashes can be relieved with cold compresses or cool oatmeal baths. Hot baths or showers may just make itching worse.
- Diphenhydramine (Benadryl) or hydroxyzine (Atarax or Vistaril) are very effective fast-acting antihistamines. Steroid creams can help keep reactions localized.

Allergies to Insects

Playing outside is one of the greatest parts of childhood, and your children should be outdoors. A good-sized welt at the site of an insect sting isn't pleasant, but it's par for the course for many people, and neither parents nor kids should be unduly alarmed. Most kids are not allergic to insect stings, even if they are prone to allergies. Nonetheless, severe reactions do occasionally occur, and it is estimated that in the United States there are at least forty deaths per year that result from insect stings.

The most common stinging insects in the United States are yellow jackets, hornets, wasps, and bees. Those of you living in the southern part of the country may have also heard about red or black fire ants that have become a major pain.

What Is Normal?

If your child is stung by an insect, the usual reaction is limited to redness, swelling, and mild pain at the site. Clean the area with soap and water, and apply an ice pack to help reduce swelling. Calamine lotion can relieve itching, but don't use it if the site is near your child's eyes or genitals.

Honeybees can leave stingers behind, and these should be removed because by doing so you can lessen the reaction to the sting. The best way to do this is to scrape the skin not pull at the stinger, which may result in squeezing more venom into the skin. Many people have found that scraping the area with something handy such as a credit card or even your fingernail does the trick. After removing the stinger, press a cloth soaked with cold water on the site to reduce swelling.

The sting of a fire ant causes a bump or itchy hive that re-solves in an hour or two. A fluid-filled blister may form at the site, which will gradually heal and may leave a small scar. When you clean the area, try to avoid breaking the blisters so they are less likely to become infected. Antihistamines and steroid creams or ointments may help relieve any itching. Sometimes the reaction spreads past the local area. The en-tire arm may swell after a sting on a child's forearm. These "large local reactions" can be frightening but are treated the same as a normal reaction. If swelling persists for a few days, some physicians will prescribe antihistamines and steroids.

Keep your child's fingernails short and clean to minimize the risk of infection from scratching. If insect bites become infected, the area might become redder, larger, and more swollen. Watch for red streaks or yellowish fluid formation. If you see these signs of secondary infection, speak to your pediatrician, who may prescribe an antibiotic.

INSECT STING ALLERGY

If your child is bitten or stung and develops any difficulty breathing, a hoarse voice, tongue swelling, chest tightness, or hives and itching in areas other than the site of the sting, this is potentially a very serious situation. Full-blown allergic reactions can be dangerous and require medical attention. Rarely, this may lead to anaphylaxis, with dizziness, a drop in blood pressure, and even loss of consciousness.

Key Point: *If your child has experienced an allergic reaction to an insect sting, there is a 60 percent chance that he will have a similar or worse reaction next time.*

Once your child has had a severe reaction, you'll always need to be prepared to respond to a potential emergency, though you may not always know what specific insect caused a severe allergic reaction.

TREATMENT OF INSECT STING ALLERGY

The emergency treatment of life-threatening allergic reactions (anaphylaxis) is so important, we have devoted a separate chapter to it (see Chapter 20). The key points, worth repeating, are as follows:

- If your child has an allergic reaction, discuss preparation for the future with your doctor.

- Make sure you always have an anaphylaxis
  kit with you, containing the appropriate dose
  of adrenaline (epinephrine).
- Always be certain you know how to inject
  epinephrine properly and that your supply
  hasn't expired.
- Seek immediate medical attention even if the
  reaction seems stopped with an injection of
  epinephrine. Sometimes additional doses are
  necessary.

Venom Immunotherapy

Allergy shots designed to desensitize people against insect
stings are one of the great and important advances in medicine. By administering gradually increasing doses of venom,
you can significantly reduce the risk of allergic reactions, usually within weeks or months. I urge you to bring any child who
has had an allergic reaction to an insect sting to an allergist
and discuss this possibility.

Avoiding Insect Stings

There are steps you can take to reduce the likelihood of your
child being stung while playing in your backyard:

- Remove hives or nests of any type, or hire an
  exterminator to do so.
- Water attracts insects. If there are areas where
  water tends to collect and stagnate, consider
  what can be done to remedy this problem.
- Keep garbage cans covered. There's not much
  you can do about uncovered ones at picnic sites

(other than stay away from them), but you can take care of this at home.

- If your family is eating outdoors, try to keep food covered beforehand.

As your children get older, teach them how to decrease their chances of getting stung. Here is some advice that parents and allergists often give, which kids usually ignore:

- Children should be taught to be on the alert for places where stinging insects are likely to gather. Look for yellow jacket nests in the ground and walls. Hornets and wasps like to nest in bushes, trees, and even on buildings. Remind your kids that stinging insects like to hang out around open garbage cans and exposed food at picnics.
- When playing outdoors, kids should avoid bright-colored or flowery clothing and sweet-smelling hair sprays, perfumes, and deodorants.
- Discourage your children from walking barefoot in the grass where it's possible to accidentally step on a stinging insect, a guaranteed way to get stung.
- If your child accidentally disturbs a bee's nest, they should quickly run away.
- Teach children not to swat flying insects. Show them that by being patient, insects will usually leave.
- Stinging insects like to crawl inside open soft drink cans, so don't drink directly from cans that have been left open outside. Transfer soda to a cup where no insect can feed without being seen.

INSECT REPELLENTS AND INSECTICIDES

I'm frequently asked whether insect repellents will reduce the risk of a child being stung. Insect repellents help prevent bites by mosquitoes, fleas, biting flies, chiggers, and ticks. I know of no insect repellents that work against stinging insects. However, I am always very specific about my advice on that topic: Use insect repellents sparingly. The most effective products all contain DEET (diethyltoluamide), which can be absorbed through the skin and cause harm. Read all labels and do not use any that contain a concentration of DEET that is greater than 10 percent on infants or young kids. Products with higher DEET concentrations may be appropriate if you will be in very highly infested areas, but they are rarely needed.

There are effective insecticides that can be placed around your yard to help eradicate fire ant mounds, though these may take weeks to work.

TAKE-HOME MESSAGES

- Reactions to drugs and to insect stings can be life-threatening and must be taken seriously.

- If your child seems to be having a reaction to a medicine, stop the medicine immediately.

- Call 911 if the reaction is severe, or otherwise see a doctor for a diagnosis. It's important to get an accurate diagnosis.

- If your child is allergic, obtain a medical ID bracelet that specifies the allergy.

- A person who reacts to an insect sting may have a stronger reaction next time, so it's important to pay attention to the first one.

- Visit a doctor for advice and for a prescription for an EpiPen. You or your child should carry epinephrine (adrenaline) with you to all outdoor events.

- Consider venom immunotherapy. It can be very effective.

- Use care with insect repellents. Some contain chemicals that aren't great for kids.

TWENTY

Anaphylaxis and Emergency Management of Allergic Reactions

I f you watch TV, it seems like a miracle that any-one makes it safely through childhood—it's sometimes easy to forget that most kids survive just fine. As I write this, my seventeen-year-old daughter is out with my car and my fifteen-year-old son is on a bike trip sharing the road with huge trucks, so I know about parental concerns. Parents of children who have had allergic reactions to food, insects, or drugs carry a special burden. Anaphylaxis—an acute systemic allergic reaction—is fortunately quite rare, but parents of allergic or asthmatic children can't help but worry about a life-threatening event.

Symptoms of Anaphylaxis

While symptoms can occur within seconds or minutes of exposure to an allergen, making the diagnosis easy, they may also be delayed for many hours. Symptoms can vary widely, depending on how much of the chemicals, especially histamine, are released. (Histamine and similar chemicals cause blood vessels to dilate and fluid to leak out into the tissues surrounding them.) Many organs can become involved:

- Skin is usually the first organ affected, with the development of all the usual signs of an allergic reaction: hives, itching, swelling, redness, stinging, or burning.

- Massive fluid leakage out of blood vessels can lead to a sudden drop in blood pressure. Your child may start to feel faint or light-headed, and even pass out.

- Engorgement of blood vessels leads to nasal congestion and swelling of the mouth and throat. You may notice a hoarse voice, and your child may complain of a "lump in their throat."

- Your child complains of chest tightness, shortness of breath, or wheezing.

- Swelling of blood vessels of the gastrointestinal tract may cause nausea, vomiting, bellyaches, and diarrhea. GI symptoms are very common if the reaction is to food.

Triggers of Anaphylaxis

Anaphylactic reactions can be triggered by allergens that are either swallowed, inhaled, injected, or have simply contacted the skin of someone who is highly allergic.

Foods known to have triggered anaphylaxis include peanuts, seafood, tree nuts, and rarely eggs and cow's milk (see Chapters 6 and 11). Sometimes foods alone are tolerated, but then a severe allergic reaction occurs when someone exercises after eating that particular food. Inhaled allergens often trigger asthma symptoms such as wheezing and coughing but actually rarely trigger full-fledged anaphylaxis. One exception is latex particles in kids who are highly allergic to latex (see Chapter 18). Injected triggers include insect stings (bees, hornets, wasps, yellow jackets) and drugs such as antibiotics in the penicillin family given intravenously or orally (see Chapter 19). Though rare, anaphylaxis has been reported in people immunized with vaccines that are prepared in an egg medium, such as influenza vaccine. Allergy shots can also trigger severe reactions.

Anaphylactic reactions cannot occur unless your child has previously been exposed to the particular allergen. If a child reacts to something on their first exposure, it is more likely to be a pseudoallergic reaction, which can actually be quite severe. The classic example of this are the contrast materials (dyes) injected during a variety of X-ray procedures. The treatment is the same for one of these "anaphylactoid" reactions.

Management of Anaphylaxis

If your child has had a severe allergic reaction in the past, make sure you always have injectable epinephrine available, know how to use it, and be certain it hasn't expired. Some of the common brand names are Ana-Kit, EpiPen, and EpiPen Jr. for children who weigh less than about thirty-three pounds. These are designed to be easy to self-administer or use on young children (see below). Your child should also wear a medical ID bracelet or necklace in case a problem occurs when you are not around.

Key Point: *If you suspect an anaphylactic*
reaction may be occurring, seek
immediate medical attention.

Treatment of Anaphylaxis

Epinephrine (adrenaline) can be injected either into a muscle or under the skin. Go to an emergency room even if your child improves, as additional treatment may be necessary. If an emergency room is not nearby or if you are uncertain that things are stable, call 911 or 0 (operator). Paramedics at the scene and emergency room staff may give oxygen, bronchodilators (asthma medications), and intravenous fluids.

How to Use an Epinephrine "Auto-Injector" such as EpiPen

If your child's physician prescribes an EpiPen, ask him or her to explain its use to you personally. (Brands of epinephrine other than EpiPen are available, but this one is common and easy to use.) As you'll see, there is no visible needle, which helps to keep a child calm so that you can inject them. Injection of epinephrine is really pretty painless. Afterward, your child might feel slightly jittery and their heartbeat may increase. This isn't dangerous. The steps are very simple:

- Remove the gray safety cap only when you are definitely going to use it.

- Hold the EpiPen (firmly) with the black tip against the fleshy outer portion of the thigh (don't cover the end of the EpiPen with your thumb!), regardless of where the reaction started. Don't try to inject into either the buttocks or a vein.

- It is preferable to hold the syringe directly onto skin, but you can actually give it through clothing if there isn't time or it isn't possible to remove them.

- Apply moderate pressure and hold for several seconds—count to ten. This releases the spring-activated plunger, pushing the concealed needle into your child's thigh.

- Since the needle retracts, you can safely discard the used syringe. If you could first place it in a plastic bag that would add a measure of safety.

- Seek immediate medical attention after using an epinephrine injection, since the effect may wear off after ten to twenty minutes. Your child should stay in the hospital for twelve to twenty-four hours for observation, since allergic reactions may have two phases, the immediate reaction and a late-phase reaction that can last for more than a day.

- If your child seems to be light-headed or faint, help her to lie down. If the reaction was from food, be prepared for the possibility of vomiting.

Key Point: *You can't have too many EpiPens.*

Keep one epinephrine kit with you, one at home, and leave one at school or day care. Here are some things to know about an EpiPen:

- An EpiPen should be kept at room temperature. Don't refrigerate it or leave it in the glove compartment or trunk of a hot car.

- Avoid exposing an EpiPen to light or heat. Leave it in the opaque case it comes in.

- You can inspect the liquid solution through the

case. The liquid should be clear and colorless. If it has turned brown or amber, get a new one.

- Be certain that you have gotten a new kit before its expiration date.

- If someone is having a severe allergic reaction, it is far better to inject expired epinephrine then not to inject any at all.

Accidental Injection into Fingers or Toes

People may accidentally inject epinephrine into fingers or toes, which can cause spasm of the arterial blood supply and threaten the viability of the injected digit. If this happens, make sure you tell them in the emergency room.

Traveling with Epinephrine

If you need to carry epinephrine while flying, be prepared for getting through security. Notify your airline in advance and again when you check in at the airport. Bring along a letter from your doctor, stating that self-injected epinephrine is essential, can be lifesaving, and must be available at all times. If you are traveling internationally, have the letter translated into the appropriate language.

TAKE-HOME MESSAGES

- If your child seems to be having a severe reaction, call 911 or (0) operator.

- If you have an EpiPen, inject it. Then go to an emergency room, as the effects of the epinephrine (adrenaline) will wear off and the reaction may continue.

- You can never have too many EpiPens. Check expiration dates regularly.

- If your child has had a severe reaction, she should wear a medical ID bracelet.

PART SIX:

ENJOYING LIFE

TWENTY-ONE

The Psychological Aspects
of Managing Allergies
and Asthma

arlier in the book you met Susanna, whose mother didn't permit her to go on sleepovers because she might have an asthma attack, and Rachel's parents who won't let her fly because of possible exposure to peanut particles from the snacks. Because of serious food allergies, Julie, age ten, only recently ate the first meal (at a summer day camp) that her mother had not personally fixed for her. Raymond's dad was yelling at him for not trying hard enough on the soccer field, while he was actually wheezing. When children have conditions where they can suffer life-threatening symptoms, it is only natural for a parent to worry. My goal—and the goal of all specialists—is to create a treatment plan that lets parents worry less and children grow into managing their own health conditions. After all, Mom and Dad really shouldn't go off to college with their kids.

Parents have a wide spectrum of personalities and attitudes about their children's health, and I learned long ago that I am not going to change a parent's personality. But it is a mistake some physicians make to either ignore a parent's anxiety or undervalue their emotions. It is important to recognize when parents are frightened and acknowledge it, and I know that reassurance is meaningless if you can't back it up with results.

The best way to help parents and children relax is to work hard to control the symptoms. One of the great rewards of caring for children through many years comes after finding a way to keep a child's asthma and allergies well controlled over time. Then, slowly, everyone starts to relax and breathe easy.

This is a delicate balance. With less concern about a child's health and a more relaxed attitude, families often drift away from the prescribed treatment plan, which can be dangerous. When asthma causes frequent symptoms, families tend to stay with the program, and their children stay well. When symptoms are mild, routine treatment often becomes inconsistent, and ironically, these are the patients we sometimes see in serious trouble in the emergency room. I want parents to feel relaxed enough to let their child lead a full and normal life, but I don't want them to quit worrying to the point that they no longer take the treatment program seriously.

Kids Worry, Too

Sometimes I meet kids who complain of a lot of symptoms and yet I see no objective signs of bad asthma or allergies. Early adolescence is a particularly tough time in the life of a child. Young teenagers are often very, very tuned in to their bodies and feel every ache and pain. Sometimes they complain they can't breathe, and yet when I listen, their chest is clear and their breathing is excellent. As parents, we all learn that each child is born with their own very individual personality and there is very little we can do about it. In other words, "It's them, not us." At any rate, some kids end up on more medications for a period of time than may be necessary, and every attempt to lower their medications meets with failure. Don't worry about it. With patience and time, your child will begin to feel more in control, and then it is easier to reduce their medications.

When I first started caring for Allison, age fourteen, she complained at every visit about feeling a daily "tightness in the chest." While medications helped, I had the feeling that I was giving her more than she really needed. It occurred to me that some of her asthma symptoms were really anxiety attacks. I explained to her parents that panic attacks are quite common; they are just as physical or organic as asthma and medications can help. With the help of a child psychiatrist, Allison's panic attacks were controlled, and very soon after that I was able to dramatically reduce her asthma medications.

I Believe in Taking Worries Seriously

A good general rule is to believe children. If children complain about mild asthma, it does no good to dismiss their symptoms. If you acknowledge their feelings as real but not dangerous, the child does much better. For instance, many kids and parents are very frightened by symptoms of exercise-induced asthma. I often see the relief in the eyes of both patients and parents when I say something like "You are not going to stop breathing," or "It is scary, but you are not going to drop dead."

I'm reminded of Matthew, a ten-year-old with long-standing allergies and asthma. He was referred to me because his asthma was not well controlled despite having excellent physicians who prescribed what I considered to be an excellent regimen. I believe his allergist had become convinced that Matthew exaggerated, since he would complain even when his chest sounded clear on physical examination.

I ordered a series of diagnostic tests and fiddled with his medications a bit, and I also was starting to believe that his problems were more in his head than in his chest. But remembering the rule that it is far wiser to believe kids than to disbelieve them, I continued to pursue rarer explanations. Finally I suggested we perform a bronchoscopy, a procedure that involves looking down the bronchial tubes with a long flexible tube and a video camera. Amazingly, we found an area where his windpipe narrowed high up in the neck, which turned out to be scar tissue around a piece of an old plastic toy he had choked on as a toddler. That tiny piece of plastic was down there for more than eight years! We removed the scar tissue and his asthma symptoms rapidly resolved.

Helping Children with Their Health

One of my major responsibilities is to help children take responsibility for their own health. I want kids to believe that their allergies and asthma can be controlled. It isn't always easy, but working together, we can successfully control their symptoms.

I work hard to adjust children's medical regimen to accommodate changes in their lifestyle. Is it easier to remember medications in the morning or before bed? If taking medicine before bed is a problem, perhaps the nighttime dose can be given at dinner. If they are going off to school all day, is there a way to adjust medications so they don't have to go to the school nurse? What sports, if any, are they participating in? If not, why not? How can we deal with soccer, football, track, the mile run, basketball?

I find that if parents acknowledge a child's anger and frustration at feeling different from their peers, it helps. Allowing privileges during treatment time is one measure that makes kids feel better. Consider permitting your child to watch her favorite TV show while she is taking her nebulizer. Kids also need to learn that everyone has stuff they have to deal with, even if their friends are unaware of it. In the big scheme, allergies and asthma are nowhere near the top of the list of problems that life brings.

If parents treat these issues as matter-of-fact—just part of life—so will their kids. If parents let their kids know that they feel "sorry for them," then their kids will feel sorry for themselves. Most kids are very intuitive and can handle just about any news that is presented to them. I also try to teach kids that if they are completely matter-of-fact about their medical needs, their friends will be totally understanding and supportive. Some kids soon find that one caring member of their group will fill the role of being the "reminder" or "guard dog" of the group, making it just one part of what a group deals with together.

Teaching Kids to Manage for Themselves

How do we let go? It isn't easy; every parent has to be true to themselves. As a parent of teenagers myself, I certainly don't know how to swim these shark infested waters. My best advice is not to be overly influenced by what other parents are doing. Rely on your own instincts. Just as it is difficult to know when to let your child get their driver's license or how late he can stay out at night, so, too, there is no one right answer to these other questions. When it comes to asthma and allergies, the art is to combine increasing independence with increasing responsibility. Parents have to let kids know that the more they are able to take on by themselves, the more freedom they will be given.

To help your child accept more responsibility, share information. It's amazing how many teenagers can't tell me what their medications are, what they are supposed to be taking and when. A child of ten or eleven (and some even younger) is perfectly capable of a basic understanding of her medications. As you move into the adolescent years, go to the doctor with her, but have her do the talking. While you need to be included in the instructions from the doctor, the symptoms really are hers and she needs to begin to acquire the skills to discuss health issues with a doctor.

However, because of the serious issues involved with asthma and allergies, you must remain vigilant with your adolescent and verify that she is taking her medications properly and consistently. This doesn't have to mean standing over her while she takes her medicine. You can often verify by checking medicine usage. If a child is supposed to be taking two puffs of her inhaler twice a day, that's four puffs per day, or about 120 sprays per month. Many inhalers, not coincidentally, contain about 120 sprays. So put down on your calendar to take a look at your child's inhaler each month and make sure she is using the right amount. Counting pills are even easier. Some newer devices such as Advair or Serevent diskus have a dose-counter built in, so it is very easy to figure out what is going on. If you become suspicious that inhalers or pill bottles are not emptying out at the appropriate rate, you have no choice but to take over for a while.

Your Attitude Speaks Volumes

Parental attitude about medication is very important. Let your child know how important these medicines are and she will take them seriously. If parents forget about these medications, so will their kids. Life is hectic, and both parents and kids do not want to think about this stuff all of the time. But asthma can kill. I am more concerned about parents who assume their kids are on top of things because they are "good kids" than parents who worry too much. If a child is supposed to take asthma medications every morning, then it remains the parents' responsibility to make sure that occurs. Just as parents should not pull the car away from the curb unless their children have their seat belts on, they should not let their child go to school without taking his medication.

One of the main reasons I urge regularly scheduled appointments for all kids with asthma, even those doing well, is that I am often able to uncover slips in routines that parents were unaware of. Parents are often shocked when I show kids pulmonary function tests that suggest maybe they are not always taking their medication; and I get them to admit that they miss medications two, three, or four times a week. Or instead of taking their inhalers twice a day, they really are only able to consistently remember once a day. (Mornings in most households are really a problem.)

If poor adherence to the regimen is imperiling a child's health, I sometimes recommend parents temporarily adopt a policy of DOT or "directly observed therapy." This means their kids have to swallow or inhale their medications right in front of their parents. Teenagers hate this, and usually after a brief period of time, they recognize the seriousness of the situation and develop better habits. Parents' attitudes are everything.

I like to make deals with kids, and this process is aided if parents take a step back and let their children speak for themselves. I'll try to simplify the regimen, even cut out some medicines, and contract with teenagers that in exchange for making things easier, they agree to stick to their medications. I also try to discuss any reasons why compliance is difficult. For instance, many kids hate watery nose sprays that drip down the back of their throat. If that is a problem, perhaps they can be switched to a dry nasal spray or we can find other ways to control their allergy symptoms.

As parents, we need to pick our fights. Many parents are

bothered by their child's constant nasal congestion and throat clearing, but their teenager doesn't really care. Sometimes it's just not worth the fight. Unless an adolescent perceives a benefit, they will not stick to medications.

Key Point: *As arms inspectors like to say,*
                 "Trust but verify."

Even a child with serious food allergies has to eventually manage independently. Allowing a child with severe food allergies to eat in strange places without you is really frightening, and I don't have easy answers. The child with food allergies needs to wear a medical ID bracelet (there are now a few brands) and carry an EpiPen at all times. Then—if she is old enough to be going out independently and is beyond the age when you can send a "safe" cupcake with her to a birthday party—you should discuss with your child before she goes to a party or even a restaurant what kinds of foods she may like to eat and what foods are safe. Practice with her by letting her select safe foods from a menu when the family eats at a restaurant. That way she'll gain experience for handling herself when she's not with you. Ultimately these choices must be made by your child. Calling the restaurant, caterer, or host family isn't usually practical because the person you speak to may not know all the ingredients, making the information unreliable. But try to convince your child to limit herself to simple, obvious, safe foods. A child who is allergic to nuts can safely eat a hot dog or pizza, but he should stay away from ice cream, pasta dishes, or Chinese foods.

TAKE-HOME MESSAGES

- Stay on top of your child's treatment so you have less to worry about and can relax—but don't relax totally. The partially treated child is in danger.

- When there are concerns—on the part of the parent or the child—these concerns need to be taken seriously. Be sure you're with a doctor who does so.

- Take your child's diagnosis in stride. Instill confidence in your child that she can lead a life unencumbered by her allergies or asthma, and find physicians who will help you reach this goal.

- Teach your child how to manage her health herself. As she gets older, step back a bit during doctor's visits and let her talk to her doctor herself.

TWENTY-TWO

Keeping Allergies and Asthma Under Control

Whether you've read this book cover to cover or dipped in and out of the chapters most relevant to you, I want to leave you with this important advice:

Key Point: *If your child's life is compromised by allergies or asthma, keep looking for a solution. Don't give up. It may take time to find it, but there is a plan that will work for every child.*

See a specialist if your primary care physician does not have symptoms under control and especially if your child has required hospitalization or even daily medications.

You and your child are co-scientists in this journey. Once a new medication or treatment has been taken for a period of time, reevaluate the situation. Are bothersome symptoms under control? Are there any significant side effects from medications? Is the treatment schedule simple enough to be manageable throughout the year?

Your child's opinion matters. If medicine tastes bad, that's important; if it's embarrassing to go to the nurse to use an inhaler before gym class, that's a valid complaint. If taking medicine midday means your child arrives late to the lunchroom, it may be a big deal. If a child just doesn't "feel that great," that's very important. Let your child know that his opinion will be voiced at your next doctor's appointment, and there will likely be a remedy. If your kids are involved in their care, they are much more likely to stick to the prescribed plan. Use a notebook to record both of your reactions so that you don't forget or "get used to it" by the time you see the doctor.

If you're not pleased, ask the doctor for adjustments. Don't settle! If your doctor is short with you or not responsive to your child's complaints, try another doctor. There are many, many medicines on the market today, and there's almost certainly a solution that will control your child's symptoms with a minimum of disruption to his lifestyle. Your current doctor can advise you about other asthma or allergy specialists, and other parents are always a great source of advice about specific physicians.

Once you find a treatment that works, stay in touch with the doctor. Most children with allergies and asthma should be evaluated by a specialist or their pediatrician at least twice a year. Remember, as soon as you think you have any symptoms "nailed," things are likely to change. When that happens, you need to change the plan.

Stay up to date on what's happening in the field. There are always exciting medical advances. New medications are coming out all the time, and there may soon be greater strides in the field of prevention. Your local newspaper's health section will give you the headlines, and there are numerous organizations and web sites listed in the appendix of the book. Check them out over the next few months, and bookmark the ones you find most applicable to your child's condition. You are going to be visiting the doctor regularly anyway, and it never hurts to be up to date on what is going on.

It takes a lot of time and effort to deal with the health issues of your child with allergies or asthma, but it is well worth the effort. Today's children with allergies or asthma can expect to lead full and complete lives. Over the years it has been my honor to help many kids bring their allergies and asthma under control, grow up and follow their dreams, then give me a hug and say good-bye when they no longer need me. There is no greater joy than watching our children mature into wonderful and healthy adults.

APPENDIX:

RESOURCES

Whether you have a question about latex allergy, indoor air quality, or asthma medications, the following resources may prove helpful.

ORGANIZATIONS

Allergy and Asthma Network Mothers of Asthmatics
2751 Prosperity Avenue, Suite 150
Fairfax, VA 22031
www.aanma.org
800-878-4403
> AANMA publishes a newsletter *(The Ma Report), Allergy & Asthma Health* magazine, e-news update on-line, and provides a toll-free help line and community awareness programs.

American Academy of Allergies, Asthma and Immunology
611 East Wells Street
Milwaukee, WI 53202
www.aaaai.org
Patient Information and Referral Line: 800-822-2762
> The AAAAI is the largest professional medical specialty organization representing allergists, clinical immunologists, and allied health professionals. For consumers, a searchable database is available, along with other resources. It also has a "Just for Kids" section of fun activities to help children learn about managing their allergies and asthma.

American Academy of Family Physicians (AAFP)
P.O. Box 11210
Shawnee Mission, KS 66207-1210
Toll free: 800-274-2237
Local: 913-906-6000
> Public information on allergies and asthma as well as specific advice on topics like getting rid of dust mites is available through the AAFP.

American College of Allergy, Asthma & Immunology
85 West Algonquin Road, Suite 550
Arlington Heights, IL 60005
www.allergy.mcg.edu
847-427-1200

The American College of Allergy, Asthma and Immunology provides an information and news service called Allergy, Asthma and Immunology Online.

American Lung Association
1740 Broadway
New York, NY 10019
www.lungusa.org
> The ALA provides detailed information on asthma, an asthma camp directory, data, statistics, programs, events, research publications, and support groups for adults and teens. For the nearest affiliate, call 800-LUNG-USA.

Asthma and Allergy Foundation of America (AAFA)
1233 20th Street, NW, Suite 402
Washington, DC 20036
www.aafa.org
800-7-ASTHMA (800-727-8462)
> The AAFA provides a national toll-free information line to those interested in learning more about asthma andallergies. It also provides practical information, community-based services, support, and referrals through a national network of chapters and educational support groups.

Center for Environmental Health
Centers for Disease Control and Prevention
Mail Stop F-29
4770 Buford Highway NE
Atlanta, GA 30341-3724
www.cdc.gov
800-311-3435
> This site offers information, facts, data, and statistics for asthma and many other health topics.

The Food Allergy & Anaphylaxis Network (FAAN)
10400 Eaton Place, Suite 107
Fairfax, VA 22030-2208
www.foodallergy.org
703-691-3179; 800-020-4040
> A nonprofit organization focusing on children. Its goal is to help individuals lead normal lives while following restricted diets.

Food Allergy Initiative
625 Madison Avenue, 11th floor
New York, NY 10022
www.FoodAllergyInitiative.org
212-527-5835
>This organization provides information about managing food aller-
gies and avoiding anaphylactic reactions.

Food and Drug Administration
Office of Consumer Affairs/HFE-88
5600 Fishers Lane
Rockville, MD 20857
www.fda.gov
888-INFO-FDA (888-463-6332)
>An informative site that includes facts on food, drug, and cosmetic
allergies; search "allergies."

Healthy Kids: The Key to Basics
Educational Planning for Students with Asthma and Other Chronic
Health Conditions
79 Elmore Street
Newton, MA 02159-1137
617-965-9637
>Helpful information for schools.

JAMA Asthma Information Center
American Medical Association
515 North State Street
Chicago, IL 60610
www.ama.assn.org/special/asthma
>This division of the AMA provides current articles, news, treatment in-
formation, education, support, resources, and links regarding asthma.

National Asthma Education and Prevention Program
National Heart, Lung, and Blood Institute
Information Center
P.O. Box 30105
Bethesda, MD 20824-0105
www.nhlbi.nih.gov/nhlbi/nhlbi.htm
301-251-1222
>NAEPP materials include:
>- Managing Asthma: A Guide for Schools
>- Asthma Awareness Curriculum for the Elementary Classroom
>- Asthma and Physical Activity in the School

- Making a Difference: Asthma Management in the School (video)
- Your Students with Asthma Can Be Winners, Too! (poster)

National Institute of Environmental Health Sciences (NIEHS)
111 Alexander Drive
Research Triangle Park, NC 27709
www.niehs.nih.gov
> The NIEHS has information on everything from general indoor air quality to cockroaches and their affect on people with allergies and asthma.

U.S. Environmental Protection Agency
Indoor Environments Division
401 M Street, SW (6604J)
Washington, DC 20460
202-233-9370

Indoor Air Quality Information Clearinghouse
800-438-4318
www.epa.gov/iaq

ADDITIONAL WEB RESOURCES AND CHAT & SUPPORT GROUPS

Allergy to Latex Education and Resource Team (ALERT): Local support network with contacts in more than twenty states. *www.latexallergyresources.org*

Allernet: This website is a great starting page for anything you want to know about allergies and asthma. From a pollen report complete with mold spore map to information on bee stings and food allergies, this network of sites will be particularly helpful in searching the web. *www.allernet.com.*

Ed's Track: Discussion Forum: Specifically for parents and caregivers to share concerns and experiences with their child(ren)'s asthma, whatever their age. *http://asthmatrack.org.*

Medlineplus: This website is sponsored by the U.S. National Library of Medicine and the National Institutes of Health, so it is a reliable source for all types of health information. *www.nlm.nih.gov/medlineplus*

Parents of Food Allergic Kids (POFAK): An on-line support group for parents of children with severe food allergies and anaphylaxis. *http://groups.yahoo.com/group/POFAK/*

The Pulmonology Channel: This website provides helpful information about all aspects of asthma. *www.pulmonologychannel.com*

Steve Carper's Lactose Intolerance Clearing House: A good site for lactose intolerance information. *http://ourworld.compuserve.com/homepages/stevecarper/welcome.htm*

Parents of Allergic Children (PAC): A nonprofit support group based in the Richmond, Virginia, area, it provides support and information to parents whose children suffer from allergies to foods, chemicals, and the environment. The main focus is for children with learning and/or behavior problems due to allergies and nutrition. *www.parentsofallergicchildren.org*

National Jewish Medical and Research Center: A respiratory hospital with special features for children with asthma. *www.njc.org/main.html*

| (aafa) Asthma and Allergy Foundation of America | STUDENT ASTHMA ACTION CARD | National Asthma Education and Prevention Program | EPA |

Name:_____ **Grade:**_____ **Age:**_____

Homeroom Teacher:_____ **Room:**_____

Parent/Guardian   Name:_____ **Ph: (h):**_____

              Address:_____ **Ph: (w):**_____

ID Photo

Emergency Phone Contact #1_____

                  Name   Relationship   Phone

Emergency Phone Contact #2_____

                  Name   Relationship   Phone

Physician Treating Student for Asthma:_____ **Ph:**_____

Other Physician:_____ **Ph:**_____

EMERGENCY PLAN

Emergency action is necessary when the student has symptoms such as, _____ ,

_____ , _____ or has a peak flow reading of _____

- **Steps to take during an asthma episode:**
  1. Check peak flow.
  2. Give medications as listed below. Student should respond to treatment in 15-20 minutes.
  3. Contact parent/guardian if _____
  4. Re-check peak flow.
  5. Seek emergency medical care if the student has any of the following:
     - ✔ Coughs constantly
     - ✔ No improvement 15-20 minutes after initial treatment with medication and a relative cannot be reached.
     - ✔ Peak flow of _____
     - ✔ Hard time breathing with:
       - • Chest and neck pulled in with breathing
       - • Stooped body posture
       - • Struggling or gasping
     - ✔ Trouble walking or talking
     - ✔ Stops playing and can't start activity again
     - ✔ Lips or fingernails are grey or blue

} **IF THIS HAPPENS, GET EMERGENCY HELP NOW!**

- **Emergency Asthma Medications**

Name	Amount	When to Use
1.		
2.		
3.		

See reverse for more instructions

DAILY ASTHMA MANAGEMENT PLAN

• **Identify the things which start an asthma episode (Check each that applies to the student.)**

☐ Exercise   ☐ Strong odors or fumes   ☐ Other _____
☐ Respiratory infections   ☐ Chalk dust / dust   _____
☐ Change in temperature   ☐ Carpets in the room
☐ Animals   ☐ Pollens
☐ Food _____ ☐ Molds

Comments _____

• **Control of School Environment**

(List any environmental control measures, pre-medications, and/or dietary restrictions that the student needs to prevent an asthma episode.) _____

• **Peak Flow Monitoring**

Personal Best Peak Flow number: _____

Monitoring Times: _____ _____ _____ _____

• **Daily Medication Plan**

Name	Amount	When to Use
1.		
2.		
3.		
4.		

COMMENTS / SPECIAL INSTRUCTIONS

_____

FOR INHALED MEDICATIONS

☐ I have instructed _____ in the proper way to use his/her medications. It is my professional opinion that _____ should be allowed to carry and use that medication by him/herself.

☐ It is my professional opinion that _____ should not carry his/her inhaled medication by him/herself.

_____   _____
Physician Signature   Date

_____   _____
Parent/Guardian Signature   Date

AAFA • 1233 20th Street, N.W., Suite 402 , Washington, DC 20036 • www.aafa.org • 1-800-7-ASTHMA
02/00

ACKNOWLEDGMENTS

Thanks to all of my patients and their parents who have taught me so much. There is not a day that goes by that I don't get a good laugh from the kids and learn something new at the same time. I also want to acknowledge all of the wonderful mentors and role models I've had throughout my training and professional career. I particularly want to thank the physicians and staff of the pediatric pulmonology division, with whom I have had the privilege to work for eighteen years.

No matter how long I spend with a patient and their family, there is no way to convey as much information to them as I have been able to put in this book. And though I had often thought of writing just such a book, it was Dr. Ann Engelland, an adolescent medicine specialist, who started the ball rolling.

I am grateful to agent Liza Dawson for not only finding a home for the book but also for offering helpful advice and support throughout the process. At Simon & Schuster, editor Caroline Sutton, ably assisted by Christina Duffy, has made it easy to be an author. Thank you to all three. And it goes without saying that I owe a deep debt of gratitude to Kate Kelly, my coauthor, who could have picked many other physicians but to my good fortune came to me with this project.

Finally, I want to thank my entire family for their love and unending support.

INDEX

Accolate, 231–32, 234, 258, 267, 288

AccuNeb, 240

Actifed, 307

action plan, 12–14, 76, 77, 191
  for allergic conjunctivitis, 312–15
  for allergic rhinitis, 297–312
  for anaphylaxis and severe reactions, 348–53
  for drug allergies, 335–41
  follow up visits for, 211, 251, 260
  for insect allergies, 341–46
  for skin allergies, 317–34
  treatment modifications in, 14, 75, 77
  see also allergies; *specific allergies*

action plan, asthma:
  controller regimens for, 211, 227–37, 258–59, 266–70
  decision on preventive vs. "as needed" medication for, 210, 217–18
  determining goals for, 210–16
  medication schedule for, 211, 244–49
  oral vs. inhaled medication for, 210, 219
  reliever medications for, 211, 237–41, 259
  selecting inhalation methods for, 210, 219–26
  supplements for reliever medications in, 211, 241–44

  written, 211, 249–51, 259–60
  see also asthma

Acular, 315

acupuncture, 116

Adam (patient), 209–10

additives, 60, 187, 317, 322–23, 338–39
  food allergies triggered by, 105, 107–8
  see also specific additives

ADHD treatments, 174

adrenaline, *see* epinephrine auto-injectors

Advair, 229, 234, 362

Aerobid, 229

Aerolate, 235

Afghan hounds, 152
  see also animals; dogs

African food, 185

Afrin, 308

Agriculture Department, U.S., 193

airborne allergens, 18, 44–48, 61, 254

air-conditioning, 129, 139, 140, 142, 171

airlines:
  air quality on, 200
  peanuts banned by, 7

air pollution, 27, 39, 48, 144–46

air purifiers, 134

air quality, 27, 39
  on airplanes, 200
  indoor, 128–39, 169
  Indoor Air Quality Information Clearinghouse, 374
  outdoor, 48, 142–46